THE ADOLESCENT TODAY IN MEDICINE

THE ADOLESCENT TODAY IN MEDICINE

NICOLAS ZDANOWICZ,
ANN DE BRACONIER-D' ALCANTARA,
V. DELVENNE
AND
P. EECKELEERS
EDITORS

Nova Science Publishers, Inc.
New York

For permission to use material from this book please contact us:
Telephone 631-231-7269; Fax 631-231-8175
Web Site: http://www.novapublishers.com

LIBRARY OF CONGRESS CATALOGING-IN-PUBLICATION DATA
The adolescent today in medicine / Nicolas Zdanowicz ... [et al.] (editors).
p. ; cm.
ISBN-13: 978-1-60021-764-7 (hardcover)
ISBN-10: 1-60021-764-8 (hardcover)
1. Adolescent medicine. I. Zdanowicz, Nicolas.
[DNLM: 1. Adolescent Medicine--methods. 2. Adolescent Behavior--psychology. WS 460 A2458 2007]
RJ550.A42 2007
616.00835--dc22

2007019186

Published by Nova Science Publishers, Inc. ✣ New York

CONTENTS

In: The Adolescent Today in Medicine
Editors: N. Zdanowicz, et al. pp. 1-16

ISBN: 978-1-60021-764-7

Chapter 1

ADOLESCENT'S HEALTH – INDIVIDUAL AND FAMILY

N. Zdanowicz[*]
Psychiatrist, Co-Head of psychiatric service, Cliniques universitaires
Mont-Godinne, Université Catholique de Louvain, Belgium

ABSTRACT

There is a paucity of research investigating which factors influence adolescents' health. Most research is directly guided by theories of social learning, and explores hundreds of variables such as the family and its functioning. Understanding and controlling these factors will allow us to influence youth's health behavior. This existing research also prompts us to reassess pathologies that occur during adolescence, and to consider them as deficient developments of health mechanisms. What seems most important to increase health among adolescents, is that parents negotiated a transfer of power of decisions to their children, and such negotiations entail sufficient family cohesion.

Keywords: adolescence, health, family.

INTRODUCTION

If health has not always been a popular topic of research, adolescents' health has commanded even less attention. While the first definitions of health date back to Cl. Bernard and A. Comte (Malherbe 1980) [1], the first research efforts aimed at promoting health really began in the sixties, only after the WHO had proposed a definition of health. Nowadays, the number of research investigating health in general is still appreciably lower than those examining pathologies. If the responsibility for this state of affairs should be partly attributed to the division of medicine into various subfields that each focuses on a particular organ, it

* Contact: Clinique Mont-Godinne, avenue E. Thérasse, 5530 Yvoir (Belgium) Tél : 003281423751 Fax : : 003281423753, E.mail : nicolas.zdanowicz@pscl.ucl.ac.be

should also be attributed to the difficulty of perceiving health as a distinctive and researchable entity. The interest in adolescence as a cohort in its own right, with its specific physio-psychological and pathological characteristics is still in its infancy. Somatic medicine units for adolescents are also still the exception rather than the rule, even though 70 percent of admissions in French pediatric units are adolescents up to 18 or older, and admission rates of adolescents are still rising[2]. Recently, interest in the health of young people has increased in our society because of two phenomena. On the one hand, diseases in contemporary are more related to lifestyles than before, and on the other, since medicine has improved the treatment of children, it must attend to an increased number of adolescent patients suffering from disorders that originated in infancy, and which would have previously been fatal. These two phenomena prompted the development of two relatively distinct fields of interest in the context of adolescence: prevention efforts (campaigns of risk reduction connected to life styles, and/or to health promotion), and research in health management.

Regardless of the direction research will follow, medicine will have to take parents into account:

- In prevention, it is critical that youth do not reproduce their parents' inadequate behaviors;
- In treatment, health professionals must keep in mind that they interact with patients who are no longer "submissive" children but who are not yet autonomous adults either.

Taking these two characteristics into consideration, there is an increasing interest in the various theories of social learning in the field of health and in combining them with systemic and family theories.

SOCIAL LEARNING AND HEALTH

One of the best known theories is Wallston's Multidimensional Health Locus of Control. This theory rests on Rotter's (1954) [3,4] more general theory of social learning, and on Levenson 's Multidimensional Locus of Control measuring tool.

This model which makes it possible to determine how individuals interact with their environment, social learning theory rests on six postulates and three concepts.

1. In order to study behavior it is imperative to take into account *both* individual (traits, needs, habits, motivation, etc.) and environmental factors.
2. Biological factors play a much less important role than social factors in accounting for these behaviors.
3. Personality is a whole that unfolds through the diverse experiences to which one is exposed. As individuals interact with their significant environments, they enhance their range of behaviors, and their personality becomes increasingly complex, and reaches greater unity and consistency.

4. The fourth postulate specifies the first: the study of behavior must take into account the joint action of both specific and general determinants, i.e. particular environmental and personality factors (personality traits).
5. The fifth postulate recognizes that human behaviors are always directed towards a goal (individuals endeavor to either control or avoid certain aspects of their environment), and asserts that they must be studied in light of this essential goal. In other words, human behaviors in terms of their motivations.
6. Finally, the sixth postulate rejects the idea that reinforcements alone can account for behaviors, and suggests another essential determinant, namely subject's expectations.

From these six postulates, Rotter extracts three concepts which underlie the prediction of a particular behavior among a wide range of possibilities:

1. The psychological situation
2. Reinforcement
   According to Rotter, a "reinforcement" is anything that affects the direction of a behavior. We note here that his concept of behavior exceeds its definition revolving around "reduction of needs" to include the idea of "a movement directed towards a goal." Hence, a stimulus has a reinforcing property (negative or positive) if it influences movement (positive or negative).
3. Expectation
   Expectation can be defined as the subjective expectation that a reinforcement will follow a behavior. It should be noted that an expectation is independent of the importance of the reinforcement, and is in theory only determined by the results of former subjectively comparable experiences.

Assessing these ideas, one notices that, if Rotter sees learning as the cornerstone of individual's behavioral choice, this emphasis does not preclude theories of personality, since his paradigm encompasses the individual's psychological situation in the process of social learning. Hence, when Rotter evokes reinforcements and their value, he refers to the subjective importance a person attaches to the expected result of her behavior. A first theorization of social learning suggested that the probability of a behavior in a situation related to a reinforcement depends on the individual's expectation that her behaviors will be reinforced, and the value she assigns this reinforcement.

In addition, Rotter (1976) [5] noted that some people do not establish any link between their behavior and its consequent reinforcement. This remark reveals that the effect of reinforcement is not an automatic process, but depends on the individual's perception of a causal relation between a behavior and its associated reinforcement. Following these observations, Rotter 1966, developed the concept of internal-external control. He defined the concept of external versus external control as the representation one holds of the relation between a given behavior and its following positive or negative reinforcement. It is this theoretical assumption that gave rise to the term "Locus of Control". Rotter conceives Locus of Control as a bipolar variable where control is on a continuum. One pole of this continuum represents complete externality and the second represents complete internality. His scale is thus general and one-dimensional. Soon after Rotter's contribution, various other scales measuring Locus of Control were created, and among those, Levenson's. These scales of

Locus of Control can be divided into the one-dimensional and multidimensional categories. These two categories are themselves divided into two subcategories: general and specific scales. General scales present a series of items generally referring to various life situations where specific scales measure expectations or beliefs in rather particular fields. Reacting to the abundant developments of the "Locus of control", Rotter (1975) [6] criticized the multiple interpretations which other researchers were assigning his concept and their confusion of his concept of Locus of Control with others as attributions, perceived control [7], personal control [8], individual cause [9], and powerfulness/powerlessness. These developments obviously resulted from the first alteration of his concept. Replacing the term of “place of control of reinforcements” with the term “locus of control” (location of control) presents the risk that the object of control – reinforcements – might be forgotten.

Levenson’s scales (1973) [10] include two axes: the internal and the external (*Powerful Others and Chance scales)*. The external axis is composed of two types of distinct (and not necessarily “additive”) beliefs : those resting on the idea of a world governed by chance, and those based on the idea of a world ruled by all-powerful people. For Levenson (1974) [11], these two types of beliefs must be distinguished because, if believing in the power of others does not draw aside the possibility of a concomitant control on behalf of the individual, believing in chance on the other hand seems to exclude it. If an individual perceives regularity in the actions of "resource people", s/he might think that s/he can obtain what s/he wishes through suitable actions which are relevant to them (maintenance of the relation, asking for assistance, seduction...). On the other hand, externality represented by "chance" is more easily associated with strong feelings of powerlessness. Although two-dimensional in its construction (intern-external), Levenson’s model thus exceeds this mere division between two independent types of externality. People are then situated at various degrees on each of these three dimensions, making the model three-dimensional.

Following this work, Wallston [12] developed in 1978 the MHLC, a multidimensional scale in the field of health. The scale aims at exploring self explanatory attitudes one elaborates about one’s health. Whereas some individuals think of having a personal role to play in avoiding or fighting diseases (internal perception of the "health locus of control"), others leave it to destiny or to the power of others – family members, or health professionals. In the same way, if some patients feel responsible and fully involved in their own treatment, others are more passive, and believe that only others (doctors, spouse, drug...) or chance are responsible for their health. MHLC thus includes three subscales: "Internality" (IHLC - Internal Health Locus of Control), "Others’ power" (PHLC - Powerful others Health Locus of Control), and "Chance" (CHLC - Chance Health Locus of Control). Apart from the scores in each of the above three scales, the following equation draws up the ratio of internality on externality [13]:

$$\text{RATIO (I / E)} = \frac{(\text{IHLC} \times 2)}{(\text{CHLC} + \text{PHLC})}$$

Using this equation makes it possible to obtain information of the one-dimensional nature in the specific field of health from a multidimensional factorial source of information. Finally, it is possible to establish a finer typology by establishing various profiles resulting from the combination of the initial scores on the three subscales [14].

FROM MHLC TO FAMILY

Since the theory of the MHLC was published, a tremendous number of other theories arose and allowed to highlight the importance of other variables. Among those, the theory of planned behaviors (TPB) [15] and the model of Self efficacy [16] are especially important.

The TPB is particularly interested in the intention of behavior which is determined by three types of factors:

- Attitude defined as one's general subjective evaluation of one's behavior;
- Subjective norms defined as one's personal beliefs pertaining to other meaningful determinants of one's behaviors, including social pressure;
- Perceived control over one's behavior defined as one's perception of the level of difficulty in adopting a given behavior.

The model of self-efficacy belongs to and is the basis of the theory of the "determinants of health behaviors". In this approach, motivations and activations of behaviors are explained on the basis of three modes of expectation:

- Situational expectations defined as the hopes in expected consequences (for example, susceptibility of the response to a treatment),
- Expectations from actions,
- One's perception of self-efficacy.

Comparing these two theories, Locus of Control appears to be exerting a more distal influence in the sense that it questions a locus of reinforcement of behaviors and not a behavior as such. Thus, in 1992 Wallston [17] reconsidered his model and proposed to incorporate the MHLC in a more general theory of health behaviors. According to this new theoretical model, health behaviors are a function of the value of health, of HLC and of one's perception of self-efficacy. The value of health acts as a regulator of the value of the HLC rather than as a multiplier [18] of it. It is the internal/external balance of loci of reinforcement rahter than the value of the IHLC alone, that is determining. It is thus erroneous to believe that internality instead of control is directly correlated with behavior. If such a correlation could be highlighted in young people in the case of the practice of a sport [19], or in the adoption of careful behaviors related to the risks of being infected with HIV, such results were not found systematically. Thus, pertaining to the risk of being infected with HIV, St Lawrence (1993) [20] did not find this "addition" of internality but did, on the other hand, find that having a high PHLC was associated with at risk behaviors. The difficulty of the MHLC and, more generally with these models, is that they attend mainly to cognitive variables, although health behaviors imply a series of other ones. Thus, still pertaining to the risk of being infected with HIV, the decision to wear a condom implies an influential emotional load which is or is not addressed. This variable undoubtedly accounts – at least partially – for the inconstancy of the results. Consequently, by widening the field from these three models to fourteen others, we can isolate more than 109 variables [21] which themselves combine in 6 factors:

1. Accessibility to services and health care [22];
2. Attitudes toward health care (belief in the quality and benefits of a treatment);
3. One's perception of the treated disease (example: first symptoms of cough of a smoker);
4. One's knowledge of one's disease
5. Social characteristics
6. Demographic factors

Factors 2 and 5 were particularly studied. These factors indeed include an individual cognitive dimension that was developed through socialization, and which includes health behaviors that can vary across subjects. Such a cognitive variation across subjects with the same background is obviously very interesting because if the determinants of this variance are known, they can also be influenced. Because they are hypothetically subject to change, these factors are thus a prime target to modify the attitudes of a subject. Various components of the 5th factor (social characteristics) intervene such as:

[1] Cultural values (for example in the dimension of the practice of a sport);
[2] Emotional factors in certain attitudes or counter attitudes pertaining to health (for example the relationship between obesity and stress);
[3] Personality factors [23], and, in young people, various parameters, such as self esteem or optimistic or pessimistic orientations [24];
[4] The influence of support groups; thus the patients with AIDS and benefiting from social support have a higher IHLC and a lower CHLC than those who don't benefit from social support [25,26].
[5] Peers' influence (for example smoking among teenagers).
[6] Influence of spouse or of family of origin (for example in the intensity of pain of chronic[3] cephalic migraine patients which is negatively correlated with family of origin cohesion and with the adaptability of the couple);
[7] The influence of the family (for example in the adherence of an adolescent to a treatment of detoxification from drugs according to the hope the parents invest in him/her [27]).

These social components are thus important to predict attitudes toward health, and parental interactions, in particular, seem to have a critical and above all, an early influence.

Family and Health

A great number of studies were interested in the implication of family relations in various disorders. The Parental Bonding questionnaire and the Olson's FACE III were mainly used. The PBI presents the inconvenience of taking into account the only factor of distance in family bonds. In the other hand Olson's circumplex model (1986) [28] (1991) [29] aims at assessing two dimensions (2 axes) of an ongoing relational system: cohesion and adaptability. The investigated system may be current : the couple, or the nuclear family. It can also pertain to a more historical dimension: the family of origin, and relate to the imaginary: the ideal family or couple to which the subject would like to belong. Cohesion is defined as the emotional bonds "that each member of the family develops with regard to the others". Adaptability is defined as "the ability of the marital or family system to change its power structure, the roles in the relations and their rules in response to a situation or a stressing evolution". Olson justifies the use of these two axes on the grounds that it takes into account various attempts of formalization of family dynamics by various authors (see for example table 1).

Table 1. After Olson (1986) [28]: theoretical bringing together

Auteur	Cohésion	Adaptabilité (changement)
Beaver and Voeller	Centripetal or centrifugal	Adaptability
Epstein et al	Affectivity	Control of behaviors Problem solving Roles
Gottman	Validation	Contrast
Kantor et Lehr	Affects	Power
L'Abate	Intimacy	Power
Leff et Vaughn	Distance	Problem resolution
Reiss	Coordination	Proximity

These two axes (figure 1) are divided into four gradations (two standard deviations), which produces a division in sixteen different subtypes likely to characterize a family. Moreover, three zones are put forward according to the balanced, average or extreme level of functioning. The model is thus designed in such way that for these two dimensions, "family health" is found in the median values of the two axes, namely "separate-connected" for cohesion and "structured-flexible" for adaptability (assumption of curvilinearity). "Health", in this model is thus an intermediate middle point and represents normality by balance [30,31,32]. The advantage of this system of classification is to avoid a strictly linear categorization such as the one found for example in Beavers-Timberlawn's model (1993) [33] where a single line slips from the state of pathology to the state of health. If Olson's biaxial system certainly presents an added value, it was nevertheless criticized for still being too normative, to some extent bi-normative instead of mono-normative [34].

In reaction to those critics [35], CH Reynaert et al. (1993) [36] proposed a model called "the umbrella model" which partially overcomes these problems of bi-normality. It will be however noted that more recent studies [37,38] reconsidered these data by highlighting a linear bond between health and cohesion-adaptability. Moreover, Fontaine (1985) [39] pointed out that even if Olson's FACES III proves to be a useful tool in clinical practice, it does not investigate all the dimensions of what could constitute a healthy family. He distinguishes in particular between a synchronic and a diachronic axis. The synchronic axis must be able to question not only the bonds between individuals and society but also the bonds between generations, both in a dimension of complementarity and of sufficient space left to others. Attempts were thus made to bring FACES III closer to "quality of communication" in families [40,41] or in couples [42]. The diachronic axis is that of time, representing the family's ability to evolve while continuously redefining itself.

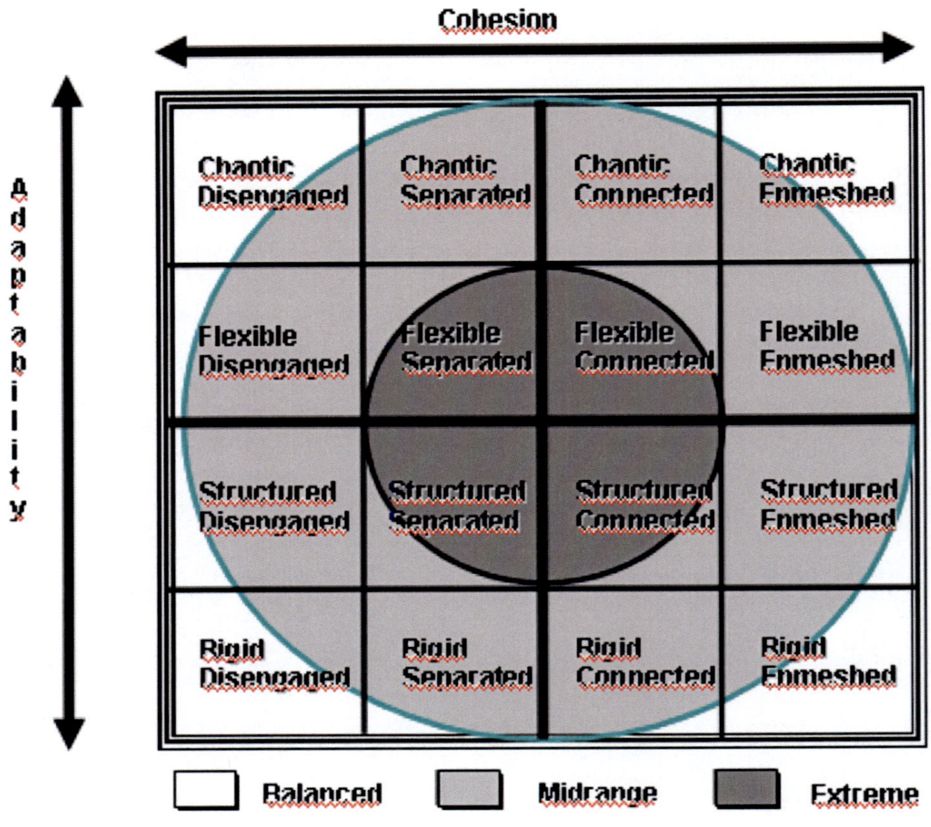

Figure 1. FACES III.

The range of the applications of FACES III is so vast that is impossible review the literature of all the fields in which it was used -- from studying the reactions of families following the stay of a child in intensive care (Youngblut 1993) [43] to the probability of relapse of schizophrenia (King 1995) [44]. Focusing on the bonds between adolescence and family, a number of studies have already investigated the relations between specific pathologies in children and young people, and family functioning (table 2). In these publications, certain nuances are necessary. Thus with regard to eating disorders, Mepherson (1996) [45] hypothesizes that family bond rather expresses itself through family dyads, and a depressive tendency (father-daughter cohesion, father-daughter adaptability, mother-father cohesion), and between depressive tendencies eating disorders. In light of all this results, Prange (1992) [46] ask if such family characteristics are a risk for a given pathology or a risk for pathologies.

Table 2. family and psychopathology in childhood and adolescence

Author	investigated issue	Age	Correlations With Olson's
Coburn and al (1989) [47]	Bulimia (B)	♀ University students	Bs belong to low cohesion families Adaptability has no influence
Ellerman and al (1995) [48]	Self esteem (SE)	5-13	SE correlated among ♂ with cohesion
Kashani and al (1995) [49]	Depression	< 13	Depressive children belong to disengaged families. Adaptability does not influence
Lawler and al (1990)[50]	Diabetes control	15-18	Diabetes control correlates with family cohesion, disengaged family presenting the worst results.
Lundholm and al (1991) [51]	Eating disorders (ED)	♀ University students	Students with ED belong to extreme families
Michaels and al (1990) [52]	Learning disorders (LD)	6-12	Children with LD belong to extreme families
Prange and al (1992) [46]	Emotional disorders (EmD)	12-18	Adolescents with ED belong to disengaged families. Poor cohesion is correlated with high rates of psychopathology.
Shields and al (1995) [53]	Delinquency (D)	Superior school students	D is associated with adaptability
Tubiana and al (1998) [54]	Diabetes control	7-13	Cohesion and adaptability are proportional to compliance to the treatment. Rigid and disengaged families = poor diabetes control
Vickers (1994) [55]	School droput (SD)	Elementary school	SD correlates with poor family cohesion and adaptability

Unfortunately, only few studies crossed the scales of health behaviors with family assessments. Apart from the studies bearing on a specific health problem in young people already cited, we found two "family" evaluations on health in general. One study (Amerikaner et al., 1994) [56] could correlate psychological health of high school students with family of origin's cohesion. The second study (Dundas, 1994) [57] showed that family of origin's cohesion and adaptability are correlated with the health of Norwegian students. But two other studies also showed the limits of tackling this issue from a single approach. May et al. (1993) [58] showed that if Olson's FACES III could be an indicator of high school students' health, it was not helpful as an indicator of a higher level of academic performance. As for him, Nagao (1999) [59], could not connect family functioning with the probability of developing a crisis of adolescence.

Although few in number [60,61,62], the studies which attempted a double approach with the MHLC and FACES III, nevertheless confirmed the existence of a correlation between family bonds and attitudes toward health. More precisely, Chirita et al. (2000) [63] could highlight that suicidal risks are not only correlated with a high PHLC but also that a high PHLC correlates with low adaptability of families of origin. Contrary to his starting assumption that hypothesized therapeutic freedom to be incompatible with too high family cohesion, Reynaert et al.. (1993) [64] showed that cohesion in the family of origin is positively correlated with the IHLC and negatively correlated with the PHLC.

Promoting Health

These various models of social learning are limited in the sense that to date, few studies have showed interest in potentially realizable cognitive changes. Indeed, if these models are to be effective, they must help us to envision strategies aiming at modifying the cognitions of an individual so that he or she would perform better in taking care of his or her own health. According to Fazio (1990) [65], there are two possible ways of modifying social determinants: one *central* and the other, *peripheral*. The central access to cognitive modifications aims at modifying cognitive data in the overall background of an individual, while the peripheral access to cognitive modifications presumes the addition of new data in favor of health. Moreover, between the introduction of new cognitive data (through peripheral or central access), and its concrete expression, a series of intermediate stages are still necessary. These stages include notions of decision, volition, and action itself. Moreover, they suppose, a dynamic mechanism in loops of retro feedback (as described by Gollwitzer, 1993) [66] which differentiates between the stages of pre-contemplation, motivation, planning, action, and maintenance. Finally, it should not be forgotten that, apart from the purely cognitive mechanisms of change, other mechanisms which are completely external to the individual can also strongly influence these choices (i.e. the relative effectiveness of anti-tobacco laws and the price of cigarettes).

Health, Family, and Adolescence: Recent Developments

Health and Today's Family

Recent research on health and adolescence highlighted various new elements of knowledge [67]:

Until now, it was thought that during adolescence, IHLC increased in parallel with the development of personality. As a matter of fact, it is *relative* internality that proved to increase with age [68]. There is no increase of *pure* internality during adolescence, which has reached the level of adult internality as early as at the age of 12, and becomes identical to it. Rather, variations in the dimensions of others' power and of locus of control are central to adolescence.

Comparisons between healthy versus "unhealthy" (presenting any disorder) teenagers suggest not only a delay of internalization of "unhealthy" adolescents both in terms of level of Internality of Health Locus of Control, and in the ratio Internality/Externality, but also more dependence on others and on chance. Furthermore, compared to healthy adolescents, "unhealthy" adolescents belong to families that were described as more "rigid-disengaged."

Apart from these correlations between teenagers' actual family and health, adolescents' health also correlates with the "ideal family" about which adolescents fantasize "for later in life" [69]. The influence of the ideal family exerts itself particularly in terms of cohesion relates to others' power. What is particularly interesting here it is that a formal thought (i.e. bearing on a non-existent object that is hoped to occur in the future - the ideal family) influences a cognitive disposition (power allotted to others), and even a biological condition (health).

Finally, dynamic links correlate age with the process of internalization of health locus of control (in particular, in terms of others' power), and family dynamics. PHLC mediates family interactions with health locus of control in the following ways:

[1] Through its decrease related to family cohesion, it initially ensures the development of relative internalization in the early stages of adolescence.

[2] But, following the above initial stage, through an increase related to the ideal family cohesion, PHLC ensures the development of at least minimal trust put in others.

Although adaptability correlates with internality, this link is less important because it doesn't seem to correlate with age. In the course of time, family (whether "ideal" or family of origin) adaptability remains as stable as IHLC.

In light of what we now know about the evolution of the Health Locus of Control during adolescence, and about family bonds, health thus seems to result from a process of reduction of the families' power over the health of their adolescent children. Attitudes toward Health, is thus not only a child's or a teenager's personal value; it is developing within the family system. This conceptualization extends both the "untying process" of adolescence theorized by the psychodynamic theoreticians, and the work of family theorists on the redistributions of roles during adolescence. If one can say that adolescence constitutes a personal crisis, it constitutes, above all, a crisis of refitting the concept of otherness, and family crisis during adolescence might be the expression of a cognitive reordering of the relative places allotted to the family of origin versus the ideal family.

Practical Implications

These results suggest several possible insights for prevention campaigns. First, these campaigns should not only concern teenagers but also their parents. Instead of being of a direct nature, (such as "Your health is your business"), the message addressed to teenagers should endorse an indirect form such as: "Health is a serious issue, don't leave it to others, chance or destiny." The message addressed to parents should invite them to disengage from their active proactive investment in the health of their children. In the same way, taking into account the findings about family dynamics, one wonders about the usefulness of a preventive campaign that would invite parents, at least in the domain of their children's health, to adopt flexible and cohesive rather than rigid and ill structured attitudes.

Detection

We might already possess diagnostic tools that enable us to forecast of both at risk behaviors, and proven pathological states. For example, based on the observation of at risk behavior, we might be able to forecast the risk of nicotine, alcoholic or other dependences in a given adolescent whom has just had his or her first experience with these substances. Confronting an obvious pathological state, an "unhealthy" adolescent involved in non rigid-unstructured family, interactive dynamics would stand a better prognosis. Such an evaluation could be followed by the establishment of therapeutic settings adapted to a determined family profile.

TREATMENT

From a therapeutic point of view we must:

- Induce parents to progressively delegate their responsibility to their children for their health;
- Remind that doctors have less chances of success when their young patients do not collaborate,
- Imperatively help an adolescent suffering from a chronic disease, to become an actively involved in actor (a subject rather than an object) his/her treatment;

Finally if the implication of a young patient to his/her treatment involves the co-evolution of his/her family system (from the cohesion and adaptability perspectives), the ideal expectations of the above young patient (in terms of ideal family dynamics) are also an important element of this evolution.

CONCLUSION

During adolescence, health is a value that evolves in the context of autonomy, and in particular, in the context of family autonomy. According to this perspective, whereas the adult paradigm defines illness as a lack in health, the adolescent paradigm perceives it as a hazard of development. This means that adolescence can be characterized by a normative process whose pathological states constitutes a failure. In the following chapters, the contributors will tackle different aspects of the interactions between health and adolescence:

Dr A. d'Alcantara : in the problems of adoption,
Dr D. Beckers : in pediatrics,
Prof V. Delvenne : in depression and attachment disorders
Prof V. Dubois: in the emergency room
Dr P. Eeckelers: in general practice
Prof C. Reynaert: in families
Dr Schepens: in problems of substance abuse

REFERENCES

[1] Malherbe J.F. Elément pour une philosophie de la médecine. *Louvain la Neuve, CIACO,* 1980

[2] Renard C. La santé des jeunes. *Bull.Educ.Patient.*2000 ; 19 : 107-109.

[3] Reynaert Ch. Pour une approche psychosomatique. Entre santé et maladie : le sentiment d'auto-maîtrise. Thèse d'agrégation de l'enseignement supérieure. Université Catholique de Louvain, Faculté de médecine, 1995. *Rotter J.B. Social learning and clinical psychology.* New-York, Prentice-Hall, Englewood Cliffs, 1954.

[4] Rotter JB. Generalized expectanties for internal versus external control of reinforcement. *Psychol. Monography.*1966; 80: 1-28.

[5] Phares E.J. Locus of Control in personnality: The Case of Karl S. New-York, General Learning Press, 1976.

[6] Rotter J.B. Some problems and misconceptions related to the construct of internal vs external control of reinforcement. *J. Consul. Clin. Psychol.* 1975; 43: 56-67.

[7] Lefcourt H.M. Locus of Control, current trends in Theory and research. Hillsdale (New Jersey), Lawrence Erlbaum Associates, 1976.

[8] DeCharms R. Personal causation. New-York, Academic Press, 1968.

[9] Reynaert Ch. Pour une approche psychosomatique. Entre santé et maladie : le sentiment d'auto-maîtrise. Thèse d'agrégation de l'enseignement supérieure. Université Catholique de Louvain, Faculté de médecine, 1995.

[10] Levenson H. Multidimensional locus of control in psychiatric patients. *J. Consul. Clin. Psychol.* 1973; 41: 397-404.

[11] Levenson H. Activism and powerful others: Distinction within the concept of internal-external control. *J. Personnality Asses.* 1974; 38: 377-383.

[12] Wallston KA., Wallston BS., De Vellis R. Development of the multidimensional health locus of control (MHLC) scale. *Health Educ. Monography.* 1978; 6: 160-170.

[13] Reynaert Ch., Janne P., Delire V., Pirard M., Randour Ph, Collard E., Installé E., Coche E, Cassiers L. From health locus of control to morphine control during patient-controlled analgesia. *Psychother. Psychosom.* 1995; 319: 1-8.

[14] Wallston KA., Wallston BS. Who's responsible for your health? The construct of health locus of control. In *Social psychology of health and illnesss.* Sanders GS, Suls J, Ed. Hillsdale (New Jersey), Lawrence Erlbaum Associates, 1982 : 65-89.

[15] Ajzen I. The theory of planned behavior. *Organiza Behav. Human Desi.* 1991 ; 50 : 179-211.

[16] Bandura A. Self efficacy : toward a unifying theory of behavioral change. *Psycholo. Rev.* 1977 ; 10 : 215-237.

[17] Wallston K.A. Hocus-pocus, the focus isn't strictly on locus : Rotter's social learning theory modified for health. *Cogn. Therapy Res.* 1992 ; 16 : 183-199.

[18] Wallston K.A. The importance of placing measures of health locus of control beliefs in a theoretical context. *Health Educa. Res.* 1991 ; 6 : 251-252.

[19] Slenker S.E., Price J.E., O'Connell J.K.Health locus of control of joggers and nonexercisers. *Percept. Motor Skills.* 1985 ; 61 : 323-328.

[20] St Lawrence J.S. African-american adolescents' knowledge, health-related attitudes, sexual behaviour and contraceptive decision : implication for the prevention of adolescent HIV infection. *J. Consul. Clinical Psychol.* 1993 ; 61 : 104-112.

[21] Cummings M.K., Becker M.H., Maile M.C. Bringing model together : an empirical approach to combining variables used to explain health actions. *J. Behav. Med.* 1980 ; 3 : 123-145.

[22] Whitehead M. The health divide. In Inequalities in health divide. Harmondswoth, Penguin,1988 : 217-356.

[23] Adler N., Matthews K. Health psychology : why do some people get sick and some stay well? *Annual. Rev. Psychol.* 1994 ; 45 : 229.

[24] Streptoe A., Wardle J., Vinck J., Tuomisto M., Holte A., Wichstrom L. Personnality and attitudes correlates of healthy and unhealthy lifestyles in young adults. *Psychol. Health.* 1994 ; 9 : 331-343.

[25] Chen M.L., Deng S.L., Chang H.K. A comparison of the health locus of control and perceived social support between cancer and AIDS patients. *Scand. J. Caring. Sc.* 2001; 15: 92-98.

[26] Fontaine K.R., McKenna L., Cheskin L.J. Support group membership and perceptions of control over health in HIV+ men. *J. Clin. Psycho.* 1997 ; 53 : 249-252.

[27] Dakof G.A., Tejeda M., Liddle H.A. Predictors of engagement in adolescent drug Abuse treatment. *J. Am. Aca. Child Adol. Psychia.* 2001, 40, 274-282.

[28] Olson D.H. Circumplex model VII : validation studies and FACES III. *Familly Process.* 1986 ; 25 : 337-351.

[29] Olson H.D. Tree-dimensional (3-D) circumplex model : theoritical and methodological adances. Minnesota, University of Minnesota 1991.

[30] Garbarino J., Sebes J., Schellenbach C. Families at risk for destructives parent-child relations in adolescences. *Child Dev.* 1985 ; 55 : 174-183.

[31] Roddick J.D., Henggler S.W., Hanson C.L. An evaluation of family adaptability and cohesion evaluation sacles (FACES) and the circumplex model. *J. Abn. Child Psychol.* 1986 ; 14 : 77-87.

[32] Benoit J.C. Dictionnaire clinique des thérapies familiales systémiques. *ESF,* Paris, 1988.

[33] Beavers W.R. Measuring family competences : the Beavers systeme model. In *Normal Family Process.* Walsch F Ed. New York, Guilford, 1993 : 73-101.

[34] Reynaert Ch., Janne P., Fontaine P., Woerlinck K., Collin A., Cassiers L. Eléments pour une reconsidération circulaire du modèle circomplexe de Olson ou : comment la logique des contraire est aussi une logique des proximités. *Thérapie Fam.* 1991 ;12 : 55-63.

[35] Steiner E., Reiter L., Klimek S. Assessing change in the course of systemic family therapy with the circumplex model by D.H. Olson et al. In *Progress in psychotherapy research.* Louvain la Neuve, Presses universitaires de Louvain, 1987 : 358-370.

[36] Reynaert Ch., Janne P., Zdanowicz N., Vause M., Vervier J.F. Description du système familial par ses membres : le sentiment d'autonomie. *Cah. Sci. Fam. Sexo.* 1993, 17 : 95-111.

[37] Smith S.G. Clinical utility of the FACES III. Dissert. Abs. Inter : Sec B : *Sci. Eng.* 1997 ; 57 : 7237.

[38] Taylor JW.V. Family structure and the coping strategies of gifted adolescents. Dissert Abs Inter: Sec A : *Huma. Soc. Sci.* 1996 :56 : 3515.
[39] Fontaine P.J. Famille saine. *Thérapie Fam* .1985 ; 6 : 267-287.
[40] Masselam V.S., Marcus R.F., Stunkard C.L. Parent adolescent communication, family functioning, and school performance. *Adolescence.* 1990 ; 25 : 725-737.
[41] Kluwin T.N., Gaustad M.G. The role of adaptability and communication in fostering cohesion in families with deaf adolescents. *Am. Annal. Deaf.* 1994 ; 139 : 329-335.
[42] Mathis R.D., Yingling L.C. Discriminant function analysis of FACES III and family satisfaction questionnaires to predict outcome in divorce mediation. *Am. J. Fam. Ther.* 1991 ; 19 : 367-377.
[43] Youngblut J.M., Shiao S.Y. Child and family reactions during and after pediatric ICU hospitalization: a pilot study. Heart-Lung. 1993 ; 22: 46-54.
[44] King S., Dixon M.J. Expressed emotion, family dynamics and symptom severity in a predictive model of social adjustment for schizophrenic young adults. *Schizo. Resea.* 1995 ; 14: 121-132.
[45] Mepherson M.A. Cohesion, conflict and adaptability within family dyads and their relations to eating disorders. *Dissert. Abst. Inter: Sec. B : Sc .Eng.* 1996 ; 56 : 7050.
[46] 46 Prange M.E., Greenbaum P.E., Silver S.E., Friedman R.M., Kutash K., Duchnowski A.J. Family functioning and psychopathology among adolescents with severe emotional disturbances. *J. Abn. Child Psychol.* 1992 ; 20: 83-102.
[47] Coburn J., Ganong L. Bulimic and non-bulimic college females' perceptions of family adaptability and family cohesion. *J. Adv. Nurs.* 1989 ; 14: 27-33.
[48] Ellerman D. A., Strahan B.J. Family functionning and children's self esteem : a test of the structure relationships of the FACES III. *J. Fam. Stud.* 1995 ; 1 : 48-57.
[49] Kashani J.H., Allan W.D., Dahlmeier J.M., Rezvani M., Reid J.C. An examination of family functioning utilizing the circumplex model in psychiatrically hospitalized children with depression. *J. Affect Disor.* 1995 ; 35: 65-73.
[50] Lawler M.K., Volk R., Viviani N., Mengel M.B. Individual and family factors impacting diabetic control in the adolescent: a preliminary study. *Maternity Child Nurs. J.* 1990 ; 19: 331-45.
[51] Lundholm J.K., Waters J.E. Dysfunctional family systems: relationships to disordered eating behaviors among university women. *J. Subs. Abuse.* 1991 ; 3: 97-106.
[52] Michaels C.R., Lewandowski L.J. Psychological adjustment and family functioning of boys with learning disabilities. *J. Learning Disab.* 1990 ; 23: 446-450.
[53] Shields G., Clark R.D. Family correlates of delinquency : cohesion and adaptability. *J. Sociol. Social. Welfare.* 1995 ; 22 : 93-106.
[54] Tubiana R.N., Moret L., Czernichow P., Chwalow J. The association of poor adherence and acute metabolic disorders with low levels of cohesion and adaptability in families with diabetic children. *Acta Paed.* 1998 ; 87: 741-746.
[55] Vickers H.S. Young children at risk : differences in family functioning. *J. Educ. Resea.* 1994 ; 87 : 262-270.
[56] Amerikaner M., Monks G., Wolf P., Thomas S. Family interaction and invdividual psychological heath. *J. Couns. Dev.* 1994 ; 72 : 614 - 620.
[57] Dundas I. The FACES III and in a Norwegian sample. *Family Process.* 1994 ; 33 : 191-202.

[58] May K.M., Logan C.R. Family type and the accomplishment of developmental tasks among college student. *J. College Stud. Dev.* 1993 ; 34 : 397-400.

[59] Nagao H. Factors that influence the ego developmental crisis state in adolescence. *Japanese journal of educational psychology.* 1999 ; 47 : 141-149.

[60] Reynaert Ch. Lieux de contrôle de l'agressivité dans les familles à transactions psychosomatiques. *Cahier. Sc. Fam. Sexol.* 1991 ; 15 : 163-172.

[61] Janne P., Reynaert Ch., de Coster P., Vause M., Cassiers L., Detry J.M., Kremer R. The spouse as a possible anginal warning system in silent myocardial ischemia. *Eur. Heart J.* 1988 ; 9 : 21-24.

[62] Janne P., du Mortier P., Mortreu B., Reynaert Ch ., Cassiers L. Matrimonio, ambiente familiare ed uclera duodenale cronica : dall'acidita familiare all'acidita gastrica. *Psicbiettivo.* 1989 ; 1 : 65-80.

[63] Chirita C., Tordeurs D., Janne P., Zdanowicz N., reynaert Ch., Roussaux J.P. La dimension familiale du processus suicidaire, une étude empirique. *Evol. Psychia.* 2000 ; 65 : 719-726.

[64] Reynaert Ch., Janne P., Vause M., Fontaine P. « Je », « nous », « vous », « eux » et « les autres ». Quelles articulations entre le sentiment d'auto-maîtrise et le vécu familial ? *Thérapie familiale.* 1993 ; 14 : 169-182.

[65] Fazio R.H. Multiple processes by wich attitudes guide behavior : the MODE model as an integrative framework. In *Advances in Experimental Social Psychology*, vol 66 Zanna M.P. Ed. San Diego, Academic Press, 1990 : 75-109.

[66] Gollwitzer P.M. Goal achievement : the role of intentions. In *European Review of Social Psychology.* vol 4. Stroebe W. and Hewstone M. Eds. Chichester, Wiley, 1993 : 141-185.

[67] Zdanowicz N., Reynaert Ch. Adolescent Health. *The Lancet.* 2004 ; 364 : 247.

[68] Zdanowicz N., Janne P., Reynaert Ch. Family, health and adolescence. *Psychosomatics.* 2004 ; 45 : 500-507.

[69] Zdanowicz N., Janne P., Reynaert Ch. Les rêves des adolescents de leur famille sont importants pour leur santé. *Ann. Méd-Psychol.* 2003 ; 161 : 190-196.

[70] Cahn R. L'adolescent dans la psychanalyse. Paris, PUF, 1998.

In: The Adolescent Today in Medicine
Editors: N. Zdanowicz, et al. pp. 17-31

ISBN: 978-1-60021-764-7

Chapter 2

THE ADOLESCENT CARE AS EXPERIENCED BY THE HOSPITAL PAEDIATRICIAN

Dominique Beckers*

Paediatric Endocrinology, Department of Paediatrics,
Cliniques universitaires Mont-Godinne,
Université Catholique de Louvain, Belgium

ABSTRACT

The aims of this chapter are to focus on the interactions between hospital paediatricians and teenagers. The consultations with in- or outpatients are the main activity of the hospital paediatrician since he sees most of the children under 16-18 years coming to the hospital. In the experience of a paediatric endocrinologist, it looks important to highlight for the practitioner how truly essential is a correct approach of the teenager and this not only because the physical changes linked to puberty have appeared but also in order to exclude any unsuspected or underlying pathology. This will allow to deliver correct informations to the patient on the normality of the pubertal development and to answer to any questions. Any source of latent anguish must be eradicated as soon as possible in the adolescent.

The basic scientific data of puberty will just be shortly recalled. More informations are easily found in medical textbooks. Case reports on the subject will be proposed and discussed.

Keywords: adolescent care, adolescence, puberty, chronic disease, functional symptoms.

* Contact: Clinique Mont-Godinne, avenue E. Thérasse, 5530 Yvoir (Belgium) Tél : 003281423462 Fax : : 003281423461, E.mail : Dominique.Beckers@pedi.ucl.ac.be

1. Introduction

Adolescence medicine has emerged in the last decades as a consequence of major scientific advances and significant societal changes related to teenagers' behaviours, and also as a result of an increase of adolescent morbidity and mortality.

As the child is growing to adolescence, the paediatrician is shifting his traditional role as advisor to the parents toward a more and more personalized relationship with the adolescent himself [1]. It is a daily challenge for the paediatrician to improve the compliance of his patient, to give him the reasons to be motivated so as to have him progressively becoming "an active actor" of his personal health care with as a final goal to preserve an healthy adult life in the future. Whatever the reason for an adolescent to be in the clinic, any risk of inadequate behavior has to be prevented.

On a daily practice, it is essential to take the time to talk with the teenager and to use the exact words to explain the objective facts or the subjective feelings. Somatic complaints often take the place of words that the teenager cannot express by himself.

Adolescence is made of major hormonal, emotional and psychological changes occurring in a relatively short period of time. Undetected difficulties during puberty may have a major impact on adolescents and their family and represent also an extraordinary challenge for all those – the family and the professionals - involved with teenagers' care.

2. Definition of Adolescence

While the beginning of adolescence is easily recognized with the appearance of signs of puberty, the end of this period is sometime more difficult to define. This sometime complicates the medical transfer of the adolescents to the internist and often, hospital or governmental rules and regulations do not help ! Nobody ends his puberty at the same age. The end of adolescence may be defined by the end of the pubertal development associated to with the development of an adult identity and the acquisition of an adult behaviour. If the first step is most of the time completed before 18 years, the achievement of the second point is clearly more difficult to assess and makes sometime the transfer to the internist somewhat difficult.

2.1. Psychological, Social and Emotional Issues

Confronted with a new developing body and new feelings, the teenagers has to learn to identify them, physically aswell as psychologically. Such an experience is sometimes uneasy to live and an external assistance is required (parents, friends or specialists). These problems will be discussed in other chapters presented in this book. Actually, the community recognizes that mental health problems as anxiety disorders, obsessive-compulsive behaviors and depression, are often present in adolescents and need special care. Even if these psychopathological problems become better understood, little progresses have been made in the prevention of teenagers' suicide, the rates of which has unfortunately remained constant for the past 40 year [2]. The understanding of the psychopharmacology of some medications for adolescents and particularly psychostimulant medications and tricyclic antidepressants has significantly improved, even if too often the methodological approach and the statistical analysis of the therapeutic results remain unsatisfactory.

After many years of practice with teenagers as a "somatician" it remains important to attentively listen to the teenagers, to develop and to maintain a mutually respectful relationship with the adolescent, to encourage the familial assistance and to praise effort to support the adolescent suffering from chronic disease [3]. Non-adherence to health regimes increases during adolescence and represents one of the challenges of the health care professional. Emotional factors, family disturbances, poor school performances and difficult peer relationships favor a poor adherence to regimes, particularly in adolescents with type 1 diabetes mellitus (TIDM) [4]. In the case of teenagers living with a chronic disease, the paediatrician has to take care of the impact of the pubertal changes affecting the evolution itself of the chronic disease and to face the specific challenges for the adolescent handicapped by a chronic disease.

2.2. Physical Issues

Puberty results from the increased secretion of sex hormones leading to the function of reproduction. Under the influence of these hormonal modifications, a fast period of growth associated to an accelerated physical transformation are responsible for the body transformation or metamorphosis.

All the teenagers worry about their physical appearance, their growth and their pubertal development. It is thus important to inform the adolescent about the pubertal "timing" especially since he may have noticed that the various morphological changes do not appear at the time he expected, this inducing some worries or even causing distress. Puberty does not start at the same time in every child.

A general rule is to be remembered There is up to a 4-years difference for the onset of puberty between the earliest children and the latest ones. Thus around the age of 12-13, some teenagers have almost finished their growth and puberty while in the same class at school, others have not yet begon their pubertal development. Provided that these normal differences are clearly explained, the teenager will be able to better understand himself. The physicians have also to make some efforts to correctly understand the links between the different pubertal stages as described by Marshall and Tanner [5] and the growth velocity . Insufficient knowledge of the problem put the family doctor in difficulties when having to decide wether the teenager has to be reassured or not. Growth and pubertal stage have to be integrated as exemplified in Appendix 1.In this table, the average age of girls and boys, the pubertal development and the age at the time of the peak of the puberty growth spurt are presented. In some cases, the radiological determination of the skeletal age represents an excellent indicator of the physiologic age and constitutes a valuable diagnostic tool for detecting pubertal abnormalities [6].

3. The out-Patient Clinic of Adolescents and the Paediatrician

Many adolescents question themselves on the normality of their body changes as they related it to their growth or pubertal development. To anticipate the questions that they not dare to raise will reduce their latent anguish and will make them trusting of his doctor.

Most of the teenagers directly consult a "somatician" paediatrician, others are secondarily referred by the child psychiatrist or the psychologists for assessing any organic disturbances which could explain the complaints. Adolescents suffering from chronic diseases, obesity or anorexia nervosa, will generally meet with the paediatric team including a paediatrician, a psychologist and quite often, a dietitian).

In the presence of his parents, the teenager will seldom express his wish to meet the doctor alone. Talking about his difficulties in the presence of his parents may raise a loyalty conflict in the adolescent's mind and some kind a feeling of betrayal towards his family. The paediatrician has the responsibility to favour a personal contact with the adolescent while preserving the parental role.

3.1. Adolescents with or without any Pathology but Having Questions about Growth and Puberty

The paediatrician has to anticipate the puberty/growth of the adolescent and has to give clear-cut explanations in due time. Almost all the teenagers worry about their developmental changes while they spontaneously remain very discreet about the delicate subject of puberty. Teenagers suffering from chronic diseases may also be concerned about their puberty, any growing delay or any other physical abnormalities.

The family doctor has to know that a 14 years-old boy who just started his puberty (testicular volume of 4 ml) will have a relatively low growth-velocity of prepubertal type (4-5 cm/year) whereas the majority of his peers will show at the same age a nice growth spurt (10 cm/year) while they already started their own puberty 2 years previously and present a more advanced pubertal stage (testicular volume of 12 ml). In this case, the patient has to be reassured and the reasons of a delayed growth linked to a late but normal puberty have to be explained (Appendix 1).

Small Height

- A 14 years-old boy is referred because of a a small height of 147 cm and because of the feeling of not growing enough rapidly while his puberty already started 3 years ago. He is indeed below the percentile 3 for his stature and his growth velocity is 4.5 cm/year while he has a testicular volume of 15 ml. There is thus a discrepancy between an adequate puberty evolution at this age and the absence of correlation with a satisfactory growth velocity acceleration. The paediatrician has to explain that this discrepancy between growth and puberty needs some investigations to rule out any hormonal or genetic problem.
- The same boy referred with the same complaints, the same height and growth velocity but with a testicular volume of 4 ml represents a different situation His

puberty has just begun 2 years after most of his peers and his growth spurt will come later in the middle of his puberty, most of his peers approaching themselves the end of their puberty and of their growth.

- A 14 years-old girl consults her physician for a small height (147 cm). However the clinical examination indicates that her pubertal development just started. This allows to formulate a good prognosis because she may expect a satisfactory period of growth forwards.
- In the case of another 14 years-old girl who comes for the same reason but who has already had her menarche one year ago, there is no much chance for further growth (on the average, the girls still take +/- 5 cm after their first menstruation).

Puberty

- A 16 years old girl worries because she has no menstruation whereas she started her breast development on time around the age of 11. If it is kept in mind that the interval between the beginning of the mammary development and the menarche averages 2 to 3 years, the teenager is justified to worry. A global assessment is required to rule out any thyroid problem, any state of hyperandrogenism or a syndrome of Turner and other endocrine or genetic disturbances.
- Another girl of the same age with the same complaint (primary amenorrhea) but who just start her breast development 6 to 12 months ago has a late puberty and no complementary investigations are needed. A clinical control over 1 year is just necessary to be sure that the puberty is correctly going on.
- A girl suffering from a Turner syndrome has to be gradually informed by her pediatrician on the risk of a non-spontaneous puberty. It will be of primary importance to propose a pubertal induction. The reasons of such a proposition have to be commented aswell as the timing and the management of the therapeutic induction. Alternatively, if the pediatrician prefers to induce the puberty later than the physiological age, the arguments should be confronted with the wishes of the adolescent.
- In a child suffering from mucoviscidosis a delayed puberty is to be expected. Preventive informations avoid any useless distress. To be recalled is that an unsatisfactory weight gain is frequently associated with a late onset of puberty. This patient will be adviced to maintain an optimal weight, a factor important to favor a normal pubertal development.

3.2. Chronic Diseases During Adolescence

Some teenagers may have their paediatrician as first referent. In second intention, they will sometimes be referred to a child psychiatrist or psychologist to help them to manage the burden of the disease. Such is the case in *T1DM*, chronic asthma, oncology disesases, Still disease, mucoviscidosis or other chronic diseases.

The prevalence of chronic diseases in adolescence is constantly increasing and the number of children with a previously fatal chronic illness still alive in adolescence has significantly raised [7-8-9-10]. For example, the median survival of patients with cystic fibrosis has doubled from 14 years-old in 1969 to 28 years in 1990 to 32 years in 2000 and more than 60% of the children diagnosed with cancer are considered as cured. Survival rates of organ transplanted children have been also improved. Eating disorders such as anorexia nervosa or bulimia have increased [11-12]. The increasing prevalence of obesity in adolescents, a situation which keeps dramatically increasing over the past 30 years, represents also a major health problem. The sedentarity lifestyle which characterizes our industrial civilisation constitutes a well recognized factor. Longstanding television watching, videogames and computer use aggravate the lack of physical exercices and the consumption of high caloric-fat diets [13-14].

Most of the ambulatory centres for teenagers have a team of paediatricians, psychologists and nutritionists working altogether. Such organization allows to integrate the various but complex and interconnected aspects of the problems during adolescence. Chronic disorders are of particular importance since they affect all the developmental issues of the adolescent life, as the relations with peers, school and education, nutrition, entertainments, projects for the future. All this represents an additional burden for them. The physicians have to help their patients to integrate their disease in their personal life. The experience of diabetes mellitus management in teenagers recently reviewed by Cameron [3] corresponds very well to our own experience in Belgium.

Example 1

- A 12 years-old girl presents a type 1 diabetes since the age of 3. She goes now to secondary school and therefore, she does not regularly make her glycemic control at noontime and follows less and less correctly her diet. Throughout the paediatric consultation, her difficulties to control her diabetes at school is emerging. The therapeutic management is aggravated by the fear of looking different from the others and the anxiety resulting from the general attitude of her schoolmates and from what they may think about her disease. A psychological guidance by a child psychiatrist or psychologist from the diabetic team is to be proposed. The goal will be to help the patient to accept and to understand his diabetic status and thus to quietly grow while coping with the disease instead of behaving as if the disease was not real.
- In Belgium, there is the possibility for all the diabetics under 18 years to benefit from a diabetic educator going to the school It is also of great importance to inform the professor and the other students over diabetes and to explain the guidelines to be respected for the treatment. It will also be worth to discuss with the professor and the teenager the difficulties encountered in his daily treatment and how its management can be improved.
- A diabetic adolescent girl is more at risk to develop overweight than the non-diabetic teenagers of the same age. Explaining the reasons of such difference and giving the appropriate informations before the beginning of the adolescence may help to prevent different problems and will avoid some feelings of culpability linked to the overweight. A non-desirable weight gain is a frequent reason for the voluntary omission of the insulin injections, this unfortunately leading to other deleterious effects consecutive to an unbalanced metabolism due to chronic hyperglycemia.

- A teenager under cyclosporine for a medullary transplant must be informed of the absolute necessity of a regular intake of his medication to avoid the rejection of the graft and at the same time about the risk of some potential side-effects like gingival[2] hypertrophy and hirsutism. Advices for a correct dental care will prevent any oral problems. If the adolescent knows that hirsutism will disappear at the end of therapy, his treatment adhesion will be better accepted.
- A teenager is on antihistaminic or valproate therapy. These drugs may stimulate appetite. If this is associated to bad preexistent dietary habits, there is a significant risk to develop overweight if no preventive explanation is given.

As illustrated by these examples, any informations given to the adolescent on his puberty will prevent many misunderstandings and will stimulate the autonomy and adhesion of the teen-ager to the health recommendations. The responsibility of the paediatrician is to inform the teenagers on the physiologic or psychopathological process involved in this particularly life period, not only by answering or anticipating the questions but also by stimulating the autonomy and adhesion to the recommended health care program. In chronic diseases, the side-effects of some drugs may be responsible for inducing hirsutism, acne, or weight gain and thus, will influence the treatment adhesion. Again talking with patients about the risks of these possible side effects are of primary importance.

3.3. Functional Symptoms in Adolescence

Some teenagers will be for the first time in touch with the paediatrician because they observe some functional or physical symptoms. Somatisation disorders are physical symptoms unrelated to any pathological finding. These adolescents complain of fatigue, headache, abdominal pain or feeling of faintness.

The prevalence of functional complaints averages 10% of the teenagers. During this period the frequency of somatic symptoms are enhanced by the mysterious body changes. The sudden emergence of the puberty transformation modifies the points of reference of the body image. This situation can induce worries and anguish when all the reference are missing. It becomes uneasy to discuss the situation. These symptoms of awkwardness shows indeed an attempt to communicate rather than a real organic problem. In some families, the body language is used as a way to communicate [15]

The physical examination of the patient is of primary importance because it gives priority to relational moments allowing to talk about the pubertal changes, the physical feelings or the psychological distress. It is essential for the teenager to have the practitioner detailing and commenting his observations, putting in simple words his appreciation of the situation. The spontaneous comments made by the adolescent should not be overlooked because they are part of their daily concern. A bodily normality is an omnipresent anxiety. Discussing bodily abnormalities implies to be able to explain the causes and possibly, to propose an appropriate health care management. Absence of fluctuations of the symptoms, absence of effect of the treatment, multiple complaints and overmedications are indicators of functional complaints [16]. While some adolescents are hospitalized for their functional symptoms, most of them have their follow-up at the outpatient clinic. If possible, the paediatrician should try to avoid an hospitalization, this attitude delivering a message of good health to the adolescent and justifying the decision of ambulatory care.

Example 2

- A 14 years-old boy presents himself at the outpatient clinic for the first time because of feeling of faintness. He is referred to the paediatric endocrinologist to appreciate a diagnosic hypothesis of hypoglycaemia. There is no particular medical or familial history apart from some social difficulties with his peers. Even if the paediatrician has no reason to suspect a very rare case of hyperinsulinism, a glucose home monitoring will be proposed symptoms of hypoglycemia appear, asking the teenager to do it during 2 weeks and to bring back the results for discussion. If upon return all the glycaemia are normal, the diagnosis of hypoglycaemia is excluded as an explanation for the feelings of faintness. "The door is now open" for another discussion on the background of the functional symptoms! If he and his parents agree on the absence of any organic problem, a consultation with a psychologist will generally be well accepted.

3.4 Personal Experience at the Paediatric out-Patients Clinic for Eating Disorders

Eating disorders in adolescents and young adults remains a serious cause of morbidity and mortality in adolescents. The pathophysiology and management of these disorders continues to evolve but research on this field is still needed to approach the best way of treatment. The following paragraphs on obesity and anorexia nervosa are based on our day-to-day personal experience with the adolescents.

3.4.1. Obesity

Since the prevalence of obesity among children and adolescents is steadily increasing (11 to 14), the hospital paediatrician is more and more often confronted with the psychological and metabolic problems associated to obesity. An endocrinopathy is rarely diagnosed but most of the parents are convinced that the obesity is not of exogenous origin but results from an hypothetical hormonal problem. After listening to the teenager and his family, it will be a priority for the paediatrician to persuade them that it is indeed an exogenous problem! When agreed by the adolescent and his parents, it will be possible to talk about diet, sport and psychological or environmental explanations responsible for the overweight.

To proceed progressively, several steps have to be systematically followed:

3.4.1.1. Anamnesis

Some questions are of interest at the first visit of the adolescent:

1) Why did you decide to take a consultation ? What is your motivation ?.

To be able to tell the doctor why he/she decided to get an advice is an indication that the adolescent wants to be active and cooperating to solve the difficulties he faces. This information indicates that the adolescent feels responsible for himself. If he is not able to explain the reasons of his presence, there is a strong indication that he has been forced to come by his parents and that it will take some time to obtain an objective approach of the situation not only with him but also with his parents.

2) Have you decided by yourself to consult with a doctor or were you not interested to come but you did it under the pressure of your parents ?

For the paediatrician, it is essential to know wether the adolescent will answer that he does "not at all", "a little" or "very much" want to take himself in charge his problem of overweight or that this is just the wish of the parents ? In this latter case, the prognosis of success is pretty low. One has to convince him that the time when he was just parents-dependent is over and that now, he becomes the main actor of his own life.

3) What is your willingness to do something for your weight problem ?

It is crucial to understand the reasons why the adolescent has taken the responsibility of taking control of his health conditions. Such informations are of great help to stimulate and to sustain his efforts. The most frequent stimuli are very simple events of the social life as the mocking jokes or the friends' glances, the anxiety of not finding a boy- or girl-friend or the difficulty of finding clothes to be nicely dressed. The idea of preventing health problems in the future or of being better in sport is less usual.

4) Do you know why you get overweight ?

Do the parents worry about a possible sickness or do they understand why their adolescent gets fat ? In many instances, the medical history and the clinical examination allow to confirm the exogenous causes of the overweight and to exclude any endocrine disorder. Complementary investigations are rarely necessary although the paediatrician has not to hesitate to ask for complementary blood investigations if he observes a reluctant attitude from the adolescent or from his parents. As long as this is not solved, no positive attitude will be obtained, particularly to modify the alimentary habits and the insufficient physical expenditures. In fifty percent of the cases, the teenager remains silent or discretely smiles when the parents confess their failure to understand the situation.

The next step is to review the personal and familial history and the endocrine or metabolic aspects involved. The growth chart is drawn. In many cases, the parents believe that the problem is just one-year old while the problem may have started at the time of the nursery school.

The dietary habits are discussed. The importance of increasing the proportion of the fruits and legumes is stressed aswell as the drastic reduction of the sugar (soft drinks,...) and the fat intake. A pleasant and tasteful health regime is proposed and the idea of "being on diet" dropped. The adolescents is warned on the false advertisements on miraculous diets as announced in magazines or in the TV advertisements. The meals timetable has to be defined and respected. Not feeling hungry does not justify missing a meal. It will be pointed out that the caloric intake has not to be too restrictive. Preventive informations will be given on anorexia. The importance of physical expenditure are stressed. The teenager will be asked to have 2-3 hours of physical activities and sport outside the school program and preferably in a pleasant and stimulating atmosphere. It will also be explained that in case of a severe stage of obesity, those having for the same body mass index (BMI) regular physical exercices are expected to have less medical complications than those who remain sedentary. Last but not least, it is to be pointed out that the personal and intrinsic qualities of an overweight adolescent have no relationship with his weight problem and that the perception of "feeling good" is not linked to the ideal weight related to the height that one could dream about.

3.4.1.2. Clinical Examination

Most of the time a good clinical examination is sufficient to rule out an endocrinopathy (thyroid disease with goiter, Cushing disease with moon facies and hypertension, syndrome with dysmorphy, a metabolic problem (hypertension, acanthosis nigricans with insulin resistance), an hyperandrogenism in adolescent girls (acne, hirsutism or irregular cycles), pseudo-gynecomastia, pseudo-micro-phallus in adolescent boys). For each of these situation, the paediatrician will explain to the adolescent the reasons of his approach or the reasons of the complementary investigations.

3.4.1.3. Discussion and Positive Propositions

The growth chart is explained to the adolescent. The normal weight related to the height is just mentioned once. While quite a number of patients and their family prefer to bury their embarrassment and their failure, the excess of weight has to be frankly commented even if this excess does not necessarily correspond to the loss of kilograms to be planned. Small but regular efforts allow to do bigger ones ! Talking too much about the ideal weight may induce a feeling of frustration. Proceeding moderately and stepwise in the reduction of the caloric intake is the best therapeutic strategy and gives the opportunity to the adolescent to be proud of himself by stabilizing his weight and=stimulates him to do better next time. Changing progressively bad habits will be much more rewarding than trying to change everything for 3 months. To be also remembered is the fact that obesity during adolescence remains quite a challenge for the future : most of these patients will continue to deal with the problem of overweight if not corrected in time. Any effort to be less fat, to eat correctly and to avoid sedentarity will preserve the health in the future of everyone. This is especially true for the obese.

In some cases of morbid obesity, it may be profitable to have the teenager being taken in charge through a dietary-oriented boarding but it is fair to drawn the attention of the adolescent that he is at risk of gaining some weight again when he will come back in his social environment. It is thus of great importance to seriously discuss the environmental problems before deciding on the boarding and not after the return in the family.

3.4.1.4. Follow-Up

Most of the cases of exogenous obesity will not be taken in charge through an hospitalization but on an out-patient basis, the child being alternatively seen by the paediatrician and the dietetician every 6-8 weeks. A psychological guidance is to be recommended but quite of number of patients or parents are rather reluctant to get the assistance of a psychologist. Owing to the growing epidemiology of obesity in children, group therapy (adolescents/parents separately) are developing. Three-hours sessions are organized including different sessions as medical and psychological consultations, dietary cooking workshops and sport. Many investigations are actually performed on the importance of different factors as the impact of the fat/sugar ratio of the diet or of the relative importance of sport versus TV and Internet.

Everyone is at risk of becoming overweight and a preventive attitude remains most important in the daily life. Efforts should be made by the family doctor and the hospital paediatrician to immediately react when overweight is noticed in a child or a teenager and this, whatever the reasons of the consultation.

3.4.2. Anorexia Nervosa

The specific aetiology of anorexia remains unclear and will not be approached here even if some indications on the role of the environment, the social factors and the psychological predisposition are available. Dieting continues to be the common entry point in both syndromes. A nice review has been published in 2003 by the American Academy of pediatrics, committee on Adolescence [11].

If the parents, the general practioner ore even the psychiatrist are worried by a constantly decreasing body mass index (B.M.I.), it becomes time to take advice from a paediatrician. He will meet the teen-ager and listen to the somatic complaints. After having completed the clinical examination, he will plot the size and weight on a standard chart and eventually propose some complementary tests. The paediatrician will then be in the right position to propose a nutritional planning associated to ponderal goals in the short, medium and long term. The paediatrician and the child psychiatrist will combine their efforts to see the adolescent from time to time but regularly in order to check how the treatment is followed and to encourage the patient.

When an adolescent suspected of anorexia asks for advice, the paediatrician may suspect that the problem has already been developing for several months. The family is overwhelmed by the situation and the family doctor or the psychologist have been of little help. In our experience, it is beneficial to see the parents when they have accepted the idea of anorexia of child and this even if the patient herself has not yet accepted and understood the problem. This last remark does not prevent meeting the teenager to check wether help or assistance is wished, to comment on her weight *vs* height and BMI and on the severity of her muscular hypotrophy. The adolescent is told that she will have no obligation to acquire the ideal weight for her height but that a too low weight can become life-dangerous, putting her body in a distressing situation as exemplified by the amenorrhea. The weight should never be less than 85% of her ideal weight nor the BMI less than 16 when the growth is over or if the adult height has been reached. Short-term objectives of reduction of weight should be defined on a 2-weeks basis. The objectives have to be constantly reassessed with the help of the doctor or the psychologist. The patient is often happy to hear that her first and immediate objective is not to get weight but to stop loosing kilos.

The adolescent should also be aware that she would be immediately hospitalized if she keeps loosing weight. Hospitalization can be made according to the hospital structures, either in the department of general paediatrics or in a specialized centre for anorectic patients, and this usually for 6 weeks. However, our policy is to immediately hospitalize if there the adolescent expresses such a wish and provided the diagnosis of anorexia is accepted. If the situation is clearly deteriorating, there is a medical obligation to hospitalize even without the patient's consent and even if the diagnosis remains unaccepted. Most of the time, the adolescent prefers to be in general paediatrics, this allowing to avoid the label of anorexia and at the same this gives a good opportunity to meet other adolescents facing different problems (diabetes type I, asthma, suicide attempts or orthopedic problems, etc…).

At the time of the first consultation, the paediatrician notes with the adolescent, her ideal weight, the weight to be reached at mid-term and the loss of weight not to be reached in order to avoid an immediate hospitalization. The first and immediate goal is to stop loosing weight rather than getting weight and this immediately within the first 2 weeks of treatment. The goal for the second period of 2 weeks will be for instance to take 500 g, etc … . In the conversation with the patient, the number of kcal/day to be taken should not be discussed in detail but rather the importance of the quality of the foods to avoid minerals or vitamins deficiencies. It is also important to explain to the adolescent that she unconsciously isolated herself from the society and as an example, that she gradually started to eat separately from the family while it is most rewarding to ~~be~~ sit altogether and to share the successes or the difficulties of the day. The same is true with her friends. Part of the therapy of anorexia is to re-integrate the patient in her normal social life.

4. The In-Patient Clinic of Adolescents and the Paediatrician

In our hospital, all the children under 18 years are hospitalized in the department of general pediatric. In all the patients, a general anamnesis of the global health status and a complete physical examination of every child or adolescent is performed, even if hospitalized for example by the orthopaedist. Adolescents general health care will be discussed, apart from the problem itself justifying the hospitalization. If necessary the paediatrician will discuss any other problem with the teenager and his/her family. This is the case for example for counselling about vaccination, allergy disease, overweight, school problems, small height, abnormal growth or puberty development, menstruation irregularity, etc… Teenagers will also be warned against some potential complications resulting from inadequate behaviours, unjustified caloric restriction, obesity, late puberty, unprotected sexual relationship, etc…

Example 3

- A teenager is developing an increasing aggressive behaviour at school and is referred to the child psychiatrist. This one observes that the adolescent suffers from the burden of his obesity and is looking for help. Since no hormonal dysfunction responsible for the overweight is found a therapeutic management essentially based on diet and physical activity will be proposed. During the physical examination of the adolescent, the paediatrician may take the opportunity to the problem of the self-image representation and some physical taboos like a small but normal penis hidden in the prepubic fat or a pseudogynecomastia related to the overweight rather to the development of the mammary gland.
- A female adolescent is hospitalized for a suicide attempt by the psychiatrist to the paediatric unit. The paediatrician is called for advice since the patient has had unprotected sexual relations with her boy-friend. The paediatrician must turn his attention to any question raised by the girl, to debate with her about contraception and also to inform her on the physiology of reproduction, the available contraceptive methods, the sexually transmitted diseases, hepatitis B, vaccinations, etc...

In these last cases, the responsibility of the paediatrician always remains to inform the teenagers on the physiological or physiopathological factors involved in this life period . He should not only answer or anticipate the questions but also stimulate the autonomy and adhesion of the adolescent as regards his health.

The physical examination is of primary importance because it gives the opportunity to talk about the pubertal changes, the physical feelings or the psychological distress. It is also very important for the teenager to have the practitioner detailing and commenting his observations, putting in simple words his appreciation of the situation. The spontaneous comments made by the adolescent should not be overlooked because they are part of his daily concern. A bodily normality is an omnipresent source of anxiety. Discussing about dysfunctions or abnormality of the body means also to be able to explain the causes and if possible, to propose an appropriate health care management.

Conclusion

Biological, physical, psychological and emotional changes are partly assumed by teenagers but require an adequate support from everyone and this not only from the family but also from the teachers, educators and friends. Undetected difficulties during puberty may have a major impact on adolescents and their family and represent also an extraordinary challenge for all those – the family and the professionals - involved with teenagers' care.

In some cases, the paediatrician has to be involved in this support. It has recently been observed a growing emergence of an "adolescent medicine" which is not only focused on "the body and the spirit" , but also on a two-steps consultation including a period of time reserved for the teenager alone different from another period in the presence of his/her parents.

References

[1] Alderman EM, Rieder J and Cohen MI. The History of Adolescent Medicine. *Pediatr. Res.* 2003 Jul;54(1):137-47.

[2] Weist MG, Ginsburg G, Shafer M. Progress in Adolescent Mental Health. *Adolesc. Med.* 1999 Feb;10(1):165-74, vii Review.

[3] Cameron FJ. *Aust. Fam. Physician.* 2006 Jun;35(6):386-90.

[4] Hauser ST et al. Adherence among children and adolescents with insulin-dependent diabetes mellitus over a four-year longitudinal follow up: II. Immediate and long term linkages with the family milieu. *J. Pediatr. Psychol.* 1990 Aug;15(4):527-42.

[5] Marshall WA, Tanner JM 1969. Variations in pattern of pubertal changes in girls. Arch Dis Child 44:291-303 and 1970. Variations in the pattern of pubertal changes in boys. *Arch. Dis. Child.* 45:13-23.)

[6] Acheson RM, Vicinius JH, Fowler GB1966 Studies in the reliability of assessing skeletal maturity from x-rays.3. Greulich-Pyle atlas and tanner-Whitehouse method contrasted. *Hum. Biol.* 38:204-218.).

[7] van dyck PC, Kogan MD, McPherson MG, Weissman GR, Newacheck PW. Prevalence and characteristics of children with special health care needs. *Arch. Pediatr. Adolesc. Med.* 2004;158:884-90.
[8] Nasr SZ. Cystic Fibrosis in adolescents and young adults. *Adolesc. Med.* 2000 Oct;11(3):589-603.
[9] Mulhern RK, Ochs J. Caring for Adolescent Cancer Curvivors: Surveillance and Intervention for Delayed Sequelae of Malignancy and Its Treatment. *Adolesc. Med.* 1994 Jun; 5(2):259-270.
[10] Ward EM, Thun MJ, Hannan LM, Jemal A. Interpreting cancer trends. *Ann. N Y Acad. Sci.* 2006 Sep;1076:29-53.
[11] American Academy of Pediatrics. Committee of Adolescence. Identifying and Treating Eating Disorders. *Pediatrics.* 2003 Jan;111(1):204-11. Review.
[12] Becker AE, Grinspoon SK, Klibanski A, Herzog DB. Eating disorders. *N. Engl. J. Med.* 1999 Apr 8;340(14):1092-1098.
[13] O'Brien SH, Holubkov R, Reis EC. Identification, Evaluation, and Management of Obesity in an Academic Primary Care Center. *Pediatrics.* 2004 Aug;114(2):e154-9.
[14] Kosti RI, Panagiotakos DB. The epidemic of obesity in children and adolescents in the world. *Cent. Eur. J. Public Health.* 2006 Dec;14(4):151-9.
[15] Caflisch M. functional symptoms in adolescents. *Arch. Pediatr.* 2005 June;12(6):811-813. Review.
[16] Silber TJ, Pao M. Somatization disorders in children and adolescents. *Pediatr. Rev.* 2003;24:255-64.

APPENDIX 1

Chronology of puberty in girls	Mean age (in years)	Normal limits (in years)
Start of growth acceleration	10.5	8 to 12.5
Start of breast development (B2)	11	8 to 13
Start of pubic hair growth (P2)	11.5	8 to 14
Start of axillary hair growth (A2)	12	
Menarche	13	10 to 16.5
End of puberty (A5 P5 M5)	15	12 to 18

Chronology of puberty in boys	Mean age (in years)	Normal limits (in years)
Start of testiculair growth 4 ml (G2)	11.5	9 to 14
Acceleration of the growth velocity	12.5	10.5 to 16
Start of pubic hair growth (P2)	12.5	10 to 15
Penis growth (G3)	13	11 to 14.5
Breaking of the voice	13.5	11 to 16
Start of axillary hair growth (A2)	14	
Appearance of the moustache	14	
End of puberty (A5 P5 G5)	15.5	14 to 18

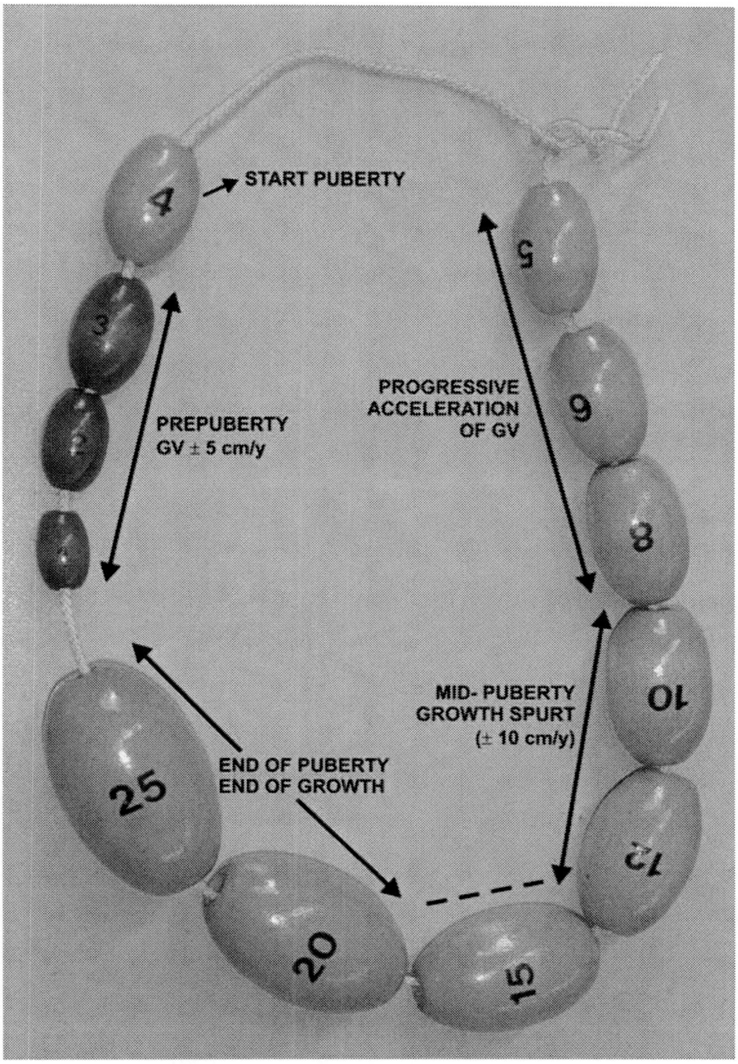

Figure. Puberty in boys : testicular volume (Prader Orchidometer) and growth velocity.

In: The Adolescent Today in Medicine
Editors: N. Zdanowicz, et al. pp. 33-49
ISBN: 978-1-60021-764-7

Chapter 3

ADOLESCENCE, HEALTH AND ADOPTION

Ann de Braconier-d'Alcantara*
Psychiatrist, Head of Centre Thérapeutique pour Adolescents,
Cliniques universitaires St Luc, Université Catholique de Louvain, Belgium

ABSTRACT

The adoption process is in and of itself a metaphor of adolescence. It is the reason why adoption situations are so explosive during adolescence, with consequences for both the physical and mental health of the protagonists.

Is it not commonly said that adolescence is a second birth, a rebirth in the sense of "Renaissance"? And, on the adopting parents side, isn't it this desire, this expectation of an "Age of Enlightenment" to come which is addressed with their adopted child, his/her future having every chance to be just gloomy, if they hadn't met at this adoption crossroads?

Adolescence on the other hand, by opening up possibilities for emancipation in relation to the governing aspects of childhood, revives both the conscious or unconscious intergenerational loyalties and therefore summons the origins, whatever is known or unknown of one's personal history.

The story of the adopted child's parents of birth, the story of the adopting parents' approach and decisions leading to the adoption as well as the story of the adoption procedure and the encounter behind the adoptive tie are all involved here.

The challenge consists of going through adolescence as a "health crisis" rather than duplicating the abandonment or breaking-off process once experienced by the child in his tie with his birth parents.

This health crisis should enable a search for one's identity along the path back towards one's origins, something that revives transgenerational determinisms, while tying them in with the adopted lineage.

The line, "sound of mind, sound of body, fit for the street" defines adolescent bio-psycho-social health.

The street updates the heartaches and pains like the love and hope words which supported the separation with the parents of birth and ended up in the adoptive filiation.

---

* Contact: Cliniques universitaires St Luc, Centre Thérapeutique pour Adolescents, ave E. Mounier 1200 Bruxelles (Belgium) Tél : 00327642002 Fax : : 00327642002, E.mail : anne.dalcantara@psme.ucl.ac.be

Keywords: adolescence, health, adoption.

1. Adoption as a Metaphor of Adolescence

If adolescence can be perceived as a second birth, couldn't adoption be understood as a rebirth-process in the sense of a true "Renaissance". And is it not so that the adoptive parents have this desire of an "Age of Enlightenment" to come about for their child whose future was bound to be gloomy if he/she could not successfully follow the path of life?

Birth, adolescence, and adoption have in common the initiatory and traumatic nature where grasping is, every time, a cutting off, a separation that will give rise to an "act of naming".

After this reshaping of ones identity, a new phase of existence begins with both continuity of the past and a break up with what has gone by, which is a phenomenon that modifies the social bond.

2. The Question of Adoption

A. Introduction

According to Alain Rey's historical dictionary, the word "adopt" would be borrowed from the juridical Latin term "adoptare" which is derived from "ad," signifying "to" or "towards," and "optare," which signifies "to choose" or "to make a choice". "To adopt" then means to choose a child through legal means. By extension, it has to do with "treating him/her as one's own child," but also" to make his/her opinion one's own," or "to chose him/her for oneself, for the long-term," or even "to approve" or "vote for [1]."

In this chapter, the word "adoption" takes us back to the situation, considered from every angle, of a child, no matter what his/her age, who has an adoptive relationship with his/her family.

The act of "adopting" is not understood to be solely restricted to a legal action. It is also a process which is comprised of numerous stages and which crosses through different levels of personal and family social life.

All these stages are important for each one of them affects the physical, mental, and relational health of the diverse protagonists in different ways, even on through diplomacy in international relations.

Situations of parental regularization of homosexual couples through adoption will not be addressed here. In effect, these new forms of parenting have not yet been around long enough to determine their effect in relation to the child who is going through adolescence.

B. Partners in the Adoption

Adoption practices go back to ancient times. They allowed for the transfer of family names, titles, and property of patrician families and most often involved the rights of young adults who had to prove something.

The stakes in the undertaking of adoption have varied over the course of the centuries. Up through the present, it has become a form of parenting that falls within the framework of national legislation, arranged by decree, and subject to agreement between countries. The Hague Convention, which was ratified in 1993, outlines the guidelines for protection of children and international adoption cooperation.

The partners in the adoption are not in a relationship of three as is evoked by the classic idea of the "adoption triangle" (the birth parents, the adoptive parents, and the child), but in a relationship of four: the birth parents, the adoptive parents, the adopted child, and a fourth group made up of adoption intermediaries, that is to say, representatives of the birth parents and governing bodies. In concrete terms, they are the orphanages and adoption agencies which are responsible for adhering to adoption laws and which lend their support to the adoption process.

Presently, all the difficulties reside in supervising the adoption situation with respect to and for the best interests of each one of these four parties.

All of them deserve equal respect in relation to that which has to do with their best interests, at first sight and emotionally, whether these interests be complementary, contradictory, and sometimes even conflictual. On one hand, it has to do with the interests of the "de-parented" child, whatever his/her condition of age, race, or health, being "unconditionally" entrusted to attentive parents. On the other hand, a couple that wants a child and has recourse to adoption defines the terms of their undertaking of the adoption process.

The conditions set forth by the adopting parents generally have to do with the age, race, and type and state of the child's physical and/or mental health.

Therefore, the concept of "adoptability" arises in relation to the child, which is not only a legal term but also defines what is considered "desirable" by the parents who are candidates to adopt.

An adoptee is both a desired child and one who is the subject of an adoption plan.

The mnemonic traces of not being wanted, a circumstance of which he/she was the object, live on in the child's unconscious and he/she will not fail to actualize it in the form of anxiety about rejection in a scenario of exclusion or projections in relation to the parental adoption plan.

For the parents, the stake will be to reconcile seeing the harmonization of the adoption plan through with their desire for a child. In effect, for a great number of them, the adoption plans are subservient to their desire for a child. Therefore, there is a kind of pressure that requires the psychological work of mourning in relation to having not been able to have one's own biological child, and finally, to accept a child born of another familial line.

The balancing out of the interests of some of the parties in relation to the others evolves within the context of the culture and can be a source of tension. Biological parents have just recently won the right to have a say in adoption matters, and presently, it mainly affects the birth mothers.

Just like the adoptive parents, they attribute their giving up of the child to circumstances that make it justifiable from their point of view. These circumstances, of course, have to do with fantasized guarantees about a future which is potentially promising and happy for the child that is given up. This mainly has to do with beliefs that give meaning to life and with the affective, educational, and socio-economic competencies of potential candidates for adoptive parenting.

The voice of these distant birth mothers deserves to be heard and considered through their narratives and the rare studies that have to do with their situation. These demonstrate just how much the giving up of their child, that they have consented to, will forever have a decisive impact on their life and just how much the unique history and grammar of this abandonment will be recorded on the child's flesh. And from this same angle, it will be recorded inside of the adoptive bond, and therefore, will negatively bias the child's possibilities for attachment to new parental figures.[3] To finally find a place, even if it is a place of lack, within the framework of the adoption process allows the adoptive parents to soothe the wounds they have suffered because of the mother being a birth mother who has lost a child.

It is amazing to note the extent to which the "progenitors" (more or less the biological fathers and/or the men present at the beginning of the child's life) are absent, as much in reality as in the discourse of everyone involved, including those who are intervening in the process. [4]

It is unusual (and only in the case of a natural disaster or war) that the biological father figures in the adoption history prior to the adoptive father coming into the picture. Consequently, the latter will enjoy a clean slate that is a priori favorable. Even so, something that has to do with the progenitor is that the mother covers herself up again in silence that attempts to make her forget his violent, degrading behavior, or his abdication of parental responsibility.

This is also an opportunity for the other partners involved in the adoption to become aware of the stakes for the child involved in searching for his/her biological roots, which is something that will punctuate the adopted children's journey through adolescence.

A fair number of these searches actually do end up as steps to reunions with initiatory trips to places of origin which, more and more, are often helped along by adoption agencies or by parent groups. [5]

Accordingly, the intermediary third part in the adoption process occupies a difficult position, one that is unanimously unpopular!

They are the consensual target of the rage that the shock of the reality of castration has for all parties involved.

Adoption is, in and of itself, an active denial of one's destiny when it is persecutory.

The end too often justifies the means, for it is during the pushing back of limits that the rescue and survival scenarios are invented.

The maintaining of ethical standards is, therefore, a particularly arduous procedure, as well as indispensable, and only an outside third party can lay claim to this duty.

It is from their place in the adoption process that the experience, tremendous potentialities, and often avoidable disappointments of so many adolescents and their parents can be harvested and made the most of for everyone.

They are also in the best position to prepare the partners for this great adventure and for ensuring preventions aimed at mental health and the frequent somatizations that occur with these children.

C. The Context of Adoption

The first step having to do with the child will be the declaration of his/her legal adoptability. This is not possible if he/she is an orphan, neglected, or if his/her biological parents have lost their rights.

Who hasn't seen the photographs, which deeply moved everyone, of those miserable, haggard, Romanian children with bulging, empty eyes, who are terrorized and starving, and are passively waiting?

Who hasn't quivered with emotion upon hearing the accounts of the fate of young Chinese girls in the foundling homes who are victims of sex discrimination? This discrimination has dangerous consequences for the gender balance of a population that 20 years later is following government measures for limiting Chinese families that desire a child to just one, without taking into consideration the cultural requirement that imposes the presence of a son at the funeral rituals of the parents. This element has caused the partial abandonment of having babies of the female sex.

Those children who have been "saved" by adoption carry in their backpack, without being aware of it, their ancestry and unique personal history.

This non-written biography passes through the context which surrounds conception and progresses up to the time of the first meeting with the adopting parents.

It carries the history of the intra-uterine life, which is so rich in experiences, passes on to birth, then the first hours of life, and finally, the time spent with the birth mother.

It carries within the unconscious the abandonment by the same, the shock of separation from the mother, the blank space. . . ., the confusion, the often long succession of intermediaries and nursemaids, over the course of time that has gone by and while waiting.

Even if this unique history will only be revealed who knows where along the thread of time and will often only be deciphered on the occasion of an existential crisis, it serves as a vehicle for the life path assigned at birth, most often by a single mother and a father in the deepest depths of an impossible genealogy. Furthermore, it conveys the drama that puts an end to their parenthood: war, death, and poverty, or shame on account of rape, incest, or a unmentionable pregnancy.

The "life debt," which is not honored by the birth parents on account of their abandonment, can only be honored by the adoptive parents if they adopt the child with their heart while recognizing his/her original lineage, that is to say, without symbolically separating him/her from his/her birth parents.

Only then does it become believable for the child that it would have been possible for the woman who brought him/her into the world to choose another mother for him/her to love, raise, and prepare him/her for life after she had conceived, carried, and grown him/her inside of her womb.

As much for the women whom life constrains from giving up their children as for the parents who are candidates to adopt, it is impossible to cover this path, with all good conscience, without the attentive presence of adoption mediators, who pass the children from one parent to the other.

The awareness of these phenomena and the considerations carried on jointly in relation to the adoption by third party intermediary partners, who are professionals from adoption agencies and orphanages, allow for the preparation of parents who are candidates to adopt and women who are pregnant, before the child is born.

This assistance allows for the accommodations for the clients, eases the suffering occasioned by abandonment, and allows for the preparation of the child for his/her future adoption.

In all of that, it is a matter of surrounding the child with "guardians of strength," that is to say, of giving him/her the tools to transform suffering into a good life experience.

Candidates who wish to adopt also benefit, in the same way, from this well-advised preparation. It does not offer them educational "prescriptions," but something beyond an awareness that will allow them to get to know themselves better and be, in their turn, "guardians of strength."

This allows parents to fully inhabit their role as adoptive parents, without erasing the child's origins, which makes them capable of a fine interpretation of the child's experience rather than feeding into their parental narcissism.

Unfortunately, this role of the adoption intermediaries is often misunderstood, or botched or boycotted by official authorities, because of the pragmatic unawareness on the part of the parents who are focused on what will happen in the short term and on the success of their plan, and finally, because of the orphan's misery that forces the adoption to clear as quickly as possible.

This support offers some additional perspectives in relation to the physical and mental health of everyone involved as well as that of the future adoptive bond.

As must be expected, it is in adolescence that this pre-history will be reactualized. The relationship between cause and effect is too tenuous for a systematic preventive policy to be practiced which would utilize knowledge acquired through experience and the social sciences.

It would not be right to fail to mention here that the field of adoption is also potentially a market that develops an "incitement" to profit from the credulity that suffering or misery confers on individuals.

This is similar to the dubious practices of illegal trafficking of human beings.

The question of health in relation to the adoptive bond is complex.

It concerns all the partners in the adoption, and therefore, also the institutional health of the adoption agencies.

The health issues of all those involved pass through procedures which are clear and obvious.

That means that institutional health has repercussions on the quality of a possible adoptive bond, based on the chances that the adoption clerk takes.

It has to do with the relational health of the teams, the ethics and competencies of the intermediaries, and the conscientiousness of all the systems that take responsibility for and prepare the children for adoption.

These cascading health effects allows for the gathering together of conditions for parental resilience upon which the quality of the reciprocal attachments between the parents and their children will depend.

These children will then, at the time of adolescence, be able to separate, differentiate themselves, and become independent, without having to repeat the emotional intensity of the moment when they were given up, along with the suffering that went along with it.

3. THE QUESTION OF ADOLESCENCE

A. What is Adolescence?

Nowadays we compare adolescence to the "social time of youth." We consider being a teenager a social reality with a social status that entails certain rights and duties.

The adolescent duty is, as well as that of any minor, that of academic obligations. And the rights are those of social participation, autonomy, and progressive emancipation, with all the responsibilities that pertain to the same.

As regards social class or age classification, the group is artificially homogenized, analyzed, and exploited, and also homoeconomicized, deciphered, and encoded.

B. Chronology

This chronological interpretation cuts the life of the young citizen into sections: childhood itself is subdivided into two distinct periods, that of young childhood which revolves around birth and school, and which is primary and tied with the mother.

Adolescence then comes about, a period of transformation which does not stop flaunting itself, from the beginning of secondary school on through the end of college, or throughout different kinds of training that entail an uncertain professional life.

Sub-periods impose themselves at this point. Some speak of "tweenage" to designate those children who experience situations where there are conflicts in anticipation of adolescence. Then there is "adulescence" to designate those young adults who hang onto the benefits derived from their socio-economic or affective dependence on the family of origin and who move past the age of thirty without taking wing.

In former times, marriage sounded the bell of departure from adolescence for young women. Military service and starting to work were the symbols of entry into the adult world for young men, an adult world that was the only one that represented "real life."

Adolescence, properly speaking, spans the time of compulsory education, between 12 and 18 years of age, and is the time when one enters the age of majority. So many times, it is taken for granted that the adolescence is not at all synonymous with being adult-like.

There are no longer any rites of passage or crises. Adolescence becomes a "slice of life" in which one is a full- fledged member.

In effect, the word "crisis," which in the Chinese language makes a link between notions of urgency and change, cannot be applied to this period called "adolescence" which has no well-defined beginning or end, and which just drifts away over the years.

Likewise, the definition of a passage is "to link one place in life to the next place in life."

If it is a matter of settling into adolescence to live one's life as a teenager, of taking advantage of one's youth, or of waiting patiently to touch down somewhere on account of a lack of initiative or because one has exhausted all of his/her resources in the world of adults, then the concept of "passage" becomes an excessive one for the adolescence.

The chronological age of adulthood finally arrives. One passes from maturity to the third stage of life, and finally on to the fourth stage of life. And doubtlessly, the generalized aging of the population will force us to open up new age categories.

C. The Adolescent Body

This chronological interpretation of adolescence is far removed from the concept of puberty which was used during the past century.

It was nubility then that was at the heart of the debate. Adolescence wasn't so much a "social time" as it was a time of bodily hormonal changes, the consequences of which lead to a reorganization of bonds.

The adolescent body confronts the subject of the feeling of oddness which is engendered by sexual urges.

The concept of "adolescence" designates the psychic operation that consists of carrying out the transformation from the infantile bond to another kind of bond so that an adult subject will come to be someone who is capable of inhabiting a body that has grown bigger and which is marked by the signs of sexual maturity, and someone who will be able to bring to his/her extended social group responsibility for what he/she says.

The explosive pubertal growth that accompanies an upsurge in hormones corresponds to an internal biological clock.

The twentieth century saw the human race grow in height by about 10 centimeters and the average age for the onset of puberty became significantly earlier, even more so for girls than for boys.

This appears in the more precocious movement towards the succession to adolescent phenomena. An article entitled, "Adolescents: The Secrets Inside Their Brains" appeared in the July issue of *Courrier International*_which knocked about the ideas that the adolescent takes in which are pertinent to cerebral maturations during the course of his/her youth.

Giedd's team has brought to the fore the important structural changes that the gray matter (composed of neurons) and the white matter (composed of nerve fibers) undergo, well beyond puberty. "If we have to settle on a new age limit for physical growth in today's humans, I would be talking roughly somewhere around 25 years of age", Giedd explains.

The adolescent speaks through his body and actions because he/she can't find the words to express so many new experiences that he/she considers incredible.

Also, this is because their emotional intensity goes beyond words. Or this might yet be because the words of childhood become inhospitable or because the boundaries of their intimate space are in the process of being completely reshaped.

This is why in adolescence one will see a new and more serious outbreak of large psychosomatic scenarios that affect sleep and digestion, and which cause back- or headaches.

Being in a more active position, young people use their bodies to express themselves inside the culture: they have their own style of clothing and they do piercing, scarring, tattoos, rasta, remodeling, etc.-I could go on and on!

D. A Specific Kind of Psychology

The question of identity appeared on the scene with intensity when the democratization of education and personal freedoms forced the issue and when the adolescent was confronted with sexuation and the failure to be responsible for him/herself. Adolescents then had to go through a process of personal psychological maturation.

This maturity, which is so necessary in the minds of contemporary citizens, was in former times reserved for a minority.

Its absence, however, was replaced by a cultural homogeneity that constituted the social bond which included the collective group.

Nowadays, this collective group is missing from the picture.

Adolescence then becomes a psychological concept and the emphasis will be placed on developmental psychology, stages of growth, the construction of personality, and modalities for intergenerational dialogue in the service of communication and education.

E. A Cultural Phenomenon [13]

There were cultural changes that adults had to confront during the second half of the twentieth century: profound reorganization of the relationship between knowledge of and the actual truth of certain situations, male/female relationships, and the bond with descendants that was henceforth programmable. All the above entail a protest, based on the authority of elders, and there is a relationship of strong opposition between the different generations.

Adolescence is set up on the front lines. It is protesting, militant, and explosive. It surrounds the social territory as if it is overtaking, step by step, the privileges of adulthood: bank accounts, an active sex life, freedom of worship, the right to have an opinion, mobility, etc.

The ambient culture is dubbed "adolescentric" and the "young look" is the model for all of society.

The paradoxical consequences are unexpected: the adult world loses its attractions, the teenagers exhibit behaviors of resistance, and denial related to the effects of growing up is seen (they are seeking to prolong the fantasy). Theirs is a flight from the painful reality associated with the daily grind, without any new rewards for adhering to it coming from the adults. And then, there's no end to searching for oneself, identified as Narcissus, in the mirror of the world. Exhilaration is followed by utter dejection . . .

What really is adolescence if it has borrowed expressions which have been so diverse over just the past few decades?

Less than a century separates us from the time when the word was not a part of our vocabulary, when the child happened upon adulthood like the young woman happened upon pregnancy at a time predetermined by her social origins.

The working class saw these little snatches away from childhood as a way for the latter to take their place in the production line while bourgeois youth were enrolled in boarding schools that had strict rules.

If neither one nor the other benefited from teenage status like contemporary youth has, they attained adult status with respect to codes and rituals which, in their respective social class, marked the steps towards maturity.

The first pair of long trousers, the first pair of nylon stockings – such were the signs of acquired privileges which echoed the restrictive duties and responsibilities of the new status.

The conclusion is forced upon us: adolescence is, before all else, a production of culture, a phenomenon.

Every historical period places an emphasis or has a particular outlook on it, expresses some facet of it, and presents it based on a predetermined mode.

It has to do with a cultural interpretation of the intergenerational report which is a recognition of a new generation, those who follow, by the preceding generation which is "in charge".

F. A Foundational Structure of Difference and Intergenerational Transmission

The symbolic order of generational succession requires that the subject is inscripted with his/her own generation and that there exists a symbolic line of demarcation that allows membership in said generation because of the difference between generations along the sequential chain that makes up the family history.

This definition advances the intergenerational bond that establishes adolescence. It no longer concentrates the weight of adolescence on just the shoulders of young people, actors in the drama and the products of change, but firmly distributes the stakes across intergenerational space.

Adolescence then is the transformation of the bond, the boomerang effect of the look that mature adults direct at youth, the effect of markers that may or may not accompany growth, the effect of the recognition of an interlocutor status which has already been registered in the transmission bestowed upon the Other, and the effect of the place recognized or shared with the Other.

Adolescence then summons up the losses (ritualized or not) proper to each generation and an awakening which is the initiation (ritualized or not) of jouissance.

This anthropological interpretation of adolescence neither minimizes nor trivializes the psychological work which is a part of adolescence.

It contextualizes it, divides it up, and relativizes it so that nowadays it leads us to excessive psychologizing and pathologizing in relation to the phenomenon of adolescence.

Therefore, it is crucial for the evaluation of any campaign that promotes overall health.

It allows for the discovery of contemporary expression that adolescents are so heavily into and determines an ideology in a tone that creates, unconsciously, new norms which are quickly and strenuously manipulated as a criterion for social inclusion or exclusion!

It is only a matter of respect that after losing ground by returning to an adolescent's unique situation one assesses, on a case-by-case basis, the upheavals occasioned by going through adolescence, i.e., the suffering, challenges, or storms of life that one runs up against, and the strengths and resources of the protagonists who are engaged in all of this.

If the subject is often nothing more than a fragile skiff on the ocean of life that is floating along on the waves of experience, its lightness, which seems so disturbing, also guarantees that it will remain floating.

4. The Adolescent in an Adoption Situation

If adoption is a metaphor for adolescence, then being in an adoption situation while going through adolescence would be a "double operation!" It summons both parents and young people, not to a repetition but a reactualization of the history and pre-history of the adoptive filiation. And this is the case for both parties (the teenager and the parents), superimposed by the symbolic going through of the birth process (with complications…), since considering adolescence as an individual's birth is something that has been agreed upon.

A. Return to One's Roots

The questions of childhood are followed by the existential questions of adolescence. [6] The "where is my life going", question stirs up the "where did I come from" question. The "who am I" question is echoed by "are my parents my real parents." "What is my place in relation to their desire?"

For the adopted child those questions pass, without fail, on to "who brought me into the world", or "why was I displaced", and "what did my parents really want." "Didn't they make a mistake?"

This last question uncovers a series of shame-inducing questions like "what if I had stayed with her," and "why did I end up with these people?".

"They are very kind and what they did was for my best interests, but in the end, they're not my real parents. So it's normal that they don't understand me. They're not the parents I was hoping to find and I think, in turn, that I am deceiving them." (Excerpt from a therapy session with Lee-Kim, 17)

To the mystery about one's origins, which often remain unknown, for many is added the enigma of why one was given up or the horror of being wrenched away from their mother. Therefore, adolescence summons up the psychological work that is necessary for the subjectivization of the separation that preceded the adoption.

For their part, the parents will take the opposite step of whole heartedness by claiming the adopted child as "our own," a whole-heartedness which forms the essence of their parenthood.

They will be confronted with certain dimensions that had been unconscious in relation to their motivations at the beginning and by the limits because of that. *"When I weigh my wife's suffering against how little gratitude our daughter shows, I sometimes ask myself if we did the right thing by leaving the Calcutta sewers. We never would have imagined that our relationship would have turned as sour as it has. If you could have seen our affectionate little girl, hanging onto her mother's knees – a real princess. Nowadays, she looks like a she-devil, all dressed in black. She's under the power of this Satanic group."* (Excerpt from a parental guidance session, because of Larissa, 16)

Lee-Kim, Larissa, and their parents are prisoners of their imaginations which maintain the idea that what *is* could have just as well *not been.* This thinking is not resistant to the relational turmoil that accompanies the changing of bonds during adolescence. The reality of daily life is not recorded in a history that can be visited at leisure, thereby putting an end to the fantasy of all that might have been.

This fantasy, reactivated by the doubts and suspicions of adolescent existential questioning, runs the risk, at all times, of repudiating the act of adoption, based on words that were offered, something which invalidates the desiring part of the adoptive filiation.

Adolescence + Adoption = rebirth + Renaissance (in the historical sense of the term)

For the young person, it is a matter of being born to him/herself and of the taking up again his/her quest in relation to his/her unknown origins with the biological parents. A tree without roots cannot stay standing when the "guardians" have moved out of the picture or when one has become separated from protective childhood figures, such as indeed are the stakes of adolescence. And in an adoption situation, these parents weren't just simply guardians providing a funnel for the young, fragile shoot, but "guardians of strength," that is to say, those who offered the child reconstructive parenting that allowed him/her to rebound from the point of an unspeakable, primordial wound, so that he/she could rediscover a sufficient amount of confidence in life to be able to dare to reform attachments.

For the parents, it is a matter of a return to the self, of questioning about the rarely explained divergence between the child's desire and the carrying out of the adoption plan at the proper time. Within this divergence, sometimes a completely non-elaborated psychological drama about an impossible "blood mother" is discovered.

The parents are confronted by surprise at the place they have bestowed upon the child's genealogical origins, most particularly, to the unconscious bond they maintain in relation to the birth mother. What scenario have they conceived of to justify the appropriation of the child to them by another woman?

Furthermore, the suffering tied in with being deprived of one's own flesh and blood mother will be revived in the adoptive mother – daughter bond when the latter becomes a woman.

By revisiting the explanatory scenario regarding the abandonment, the young person completely confronts it with the "desire for adoption," which is the carrier of his/her parents' conscious and unconscious motivations.

The words which were spoken during childhood take on all of their importance at this point.

Accepted, without calling them into question, within the trust based on the infantile bond, these words turn out to be reparatory or, and on the other hand, reassuring at the time in question. But he/she has not been able to give him/herself over to thinking through or dressing the wounds of the trauma occasioned by the loss that is superimposed on the trauma of birth.

B. The Act of Adoption and Mixed Loyalties

Thus, adolescence within an adoption situation is a particular stage which reveals the reverse side of the act of adoption.

This act is, in effect, as understood from the parents' side who adopt the child by recording him/her within a symbolic filiation through the changing of his/her civil status, a change that makes of him/her their child.

If the adoption makes them his/her parents completely, and if this adopted child becomes their child whole-heartedly, he/she does not necessarily remain the child of the biological couple, also, historically speaking.

At adolescence, the parents assess how the child has been able or has not been able to respond to the plenary act of adoption.

Several scenarios are presented, as follows:

1. Certain children remain within the legal aspect of the adoption contract. Although they appeared to be well-adapted in childhood, they seem to have "borrowed", as a replacement for the lost parents, parents whose love has nurtured them throughout their time of "immaturity" but to whom they are not attached.

Having grown bigger and longing for independence, it is as if the teenager had only treated his/her adoptive parents like his real parents without, for all of that, having to choose for him/herself in a lasting way.

In this case, is it loyalty to the biological parents that prevails when the time comes for him/her to set off on his/her own or do they consider themselves unattached survivors that have nothing to lose?

Adolescence, in these kinds of cases, is doubly conflictual within the intergenerational bond. Adolescents cannot tolerate any guidance and take risks through challenging authority, going through depression and delinquency, addictive behaviors, and taking actions that are doomed to failure. But scholastic ambitions and early emancipation can also punctuate their life path and it isn't rare for parents who have taken a short-cut for all of that to become desperate when they see their adolescents decompensate.

"Joe-Ki is the oldest of four, all of whom were born in Korea. A model child, he is very appreciated by the whole family and he is his paternal grandparents favorite. When he was fifteen, he changed drastically. Indifferent to everything, he only carries out actions in his head. He isolates himself and barks at anyone who disturbs him. His brothers and his sister, whom at first had been spared, are swept along, in their turn, inside of the tempest. Even the youngest, whom he had protected since his arrival and who is his godchild, can no longer get a smile out of him. His mother finds him unbearable and launches into violent behavior. He runs away from his father and spends most of his time somewhere else so that when he's at home, he treats it like a second-rate hotel. He only makes an appearance to ask for pocket money which he calls his "weekly pay." A failed school year as well as regular consumption of cannabis caused his parents to blow up, which was the reason for the consultation. Joe-Ki will only come in for consultation one time to say that he is an intergalactic space shuttle who is rightfully loaded up with adoptive fuel. He said that his parents make up a useless ballast tank and that they cling onto him like scotch tape, inside of a tearful Romanticism. For their part, they took the time to receive guidance throughout the time they were going through this."

A demanding overture is necessary with the parents when they become aware of their adolescent's emotional poverty in relation to his investment in the bond. This is the kind of child who will never desire to be adopted in return for the parents who are offered to him/her. He/she is a child who, in the best of cases, will content him/herself with just showing the respect due the guardian.

A lot of confidence and tenacity is often needed to get through that which could only be experienced as a misunderstanding. This misunderstanding is structurally present from the start of every adoptive encounter and is tied into the fact that the child is in a survival arrangement: his request is articulated based on a need for security which in and of itself is not a guarantee that it might be born of desire for a bond of filial love.

These noisy adolescents express the deconstruction of the dependent bond in relation to the parents. These stirrings are worth of the intensity of the experience of dependency and cannabis consumption is one representation of this.

2. On the contrary, many adoptees have been able to make their adoptive parents "really theirs." In return, both of them, or just one of the two, have "really" adopted them. This is the proof that they have transcended the narcissistic wound of the abandonment since they have found that their welcoming parents desire a child within the respect they have for their biological descendents.

They have been able to intertwine double loyalties that cross over one another in the Imaginary and the Real, without betraying either of them. They are not identified with the explanatory fantasy of their filiation, but they have succeeded in writing their history in relation to the beginning of their lives.[7]

Often this movement can only come about after intense internal turmoil which is accompanied by a rejection of his/her origins and the adoptive parents, in turn. Massive anxieties and researching traces of the past ensue.

They will be lead to a renunciation of the alienating project of reparation with both their birth and adoptive parents.

And because of abuses occasioned by life, the fact of the adoption seizes onto the same to develop the desiring and constructive potential of the bond.

"Rumi questions her future and her origins. The adoption took over its place within the narrative of her life. She mentions it like it's just another element of her history within the regression of her therapy which got underway after the break-up of a love relationship that was followed by a suicide attempt."

At the most, the issue of the adoption for this young person will create a "chamber of resonance" for the inescapable existential question that arises during the process of growth. It will create a pretext but not an alibi for his/her construction of a search for identity. Still, it is necessary that the therapist doesn't close down the issue by an interpretation couched in terms of the "non-attachment syndrome." In effect, this syndrome, which suggests that the child lacks attachment competency and which victimizes the therapeutic approach itself, if it is not called into question, runs the risk of gaining approval because of its compromising nature which is apt to exculpate all parties involved.

3. Remaining within the anguish of repetition and the terror of rejection, many adopted teenagers curl up inside of parental desire without ever daring to confront the adoption plans and facts of their pre-history.

They accepted the version that was related to them during childhood. They will continue to move along the loop line of their critical trajectory, stuck with the adoptee identity, prisoners of the adoptive parents' desire, anxious for familial homeostasis that is only achieved with difficulty.

They give up renewing their ties with the one who was inscribed before in their skin of fear because of the possibility of provoking, in their turn, the trembling of the earth that shook up the beginning of their existence.

It is this strong adolescent ambivalence, in relation to the parents, that paradoxically paralyzes them and serves as an alibi for their resignation.

C. The Life Debt

It's because the little man/woman is powerless and is totally dependent that his/her own life must be transmitted to him/her, that is to say he/she must be "humanized." This is why bringing him/her into the world at birth is accompanied by the transmission of a debt which, if it is paid out by the parents and contracted by the child, will one day be transmitted to the latter's children.

The desire to pay off this debt with the child is part of the "desire to adopt" for candidates who want to be adoptive parents. This unconscious, symbolic debt is the counterpart of the little man's/little woman's immaturity. He/she must give the debt recognition in order to contract it, before he/she can hand it down, in his/her turn.

If after a traumatic experience (because the trauma of abandonment is forever pegged to the body) the subject presents a fantasy that triggers off repetition compulsion behavior, the debt does not become symbolized since the child does not feel that he/she has been understood.[8]

During adolescence, the young adoptee will go through productions of this fantasy.

Without comprehending it, he/she will make his/her entourage see and experience the impasse that holds him/her prisoner. He/she persecutes the other about the imagined debt through projection, taking the position that "it's up to the other one to pay."

Both parents are then unable to cope. They are considered old-fashioned, hostile, and are brutally dismissed in a whirl because of unconscious motivations coming from way back.

Clinical histories that indicate mistreatment, murderous conflicts, and cruel rejection give rise to a pathological bond that provokes one to go on to the act that could lead up to a breach of the contract.

All are then obligated to dip into their previously untapped resources to appeal to third party adoption professionals or psychotherapists whose interpretations pinpoint the scenario which repeats itself, over and over again.

Becoming aware of all of this allows the protagonists to put it at a distance and reconcile themselves to their unique history.

D. One's Body

The beginnings of life

Françoise Dolto remembers us *how important it is for a subject in adolescence to totally assume the "primitive scene". It makes him possible to accept his body, his history, both lines of ascendants, or his unknown lineages. As a subject he is presentified by one's body, and if that body is accepted as well it is able to tell about his origin* [9]

Many adolescents travel trough the mirror to find trails of the lost dad or mam on their growing ,changing face, aware of the possible reading of their body linked with the origin. Lonelyness becomes the way to bound with "No-body" and to discover inside- roots.

Emotional tuning start from one's body.

Obesity, the surch of sensations and excitements, drugs, alcohol, acting out and delinquant behaviour, suïcid attempts and automutilation, but also sport performance becomes the expression of the double adolescence process [10]

5. Conclusion

Birth separates the child from the maternal body and carries out the passage of one's life from an existence surrounded by fluid to one surrounded by air.

Adoption separates a child, from his/her roots even though he/she is powerless to survive on his/her own.

Adolescence opens up perspectives on emancipation in relation to parental figures who have governed one's childhood.

At the same time, it stirs up conscious or unconscious intergenerational loyalties and therefore summons the origins, whether or not the actors are aware of or are ignorant of their history. It has to do with the adopted child's birth parents, the history of the steps that led to the other parents to adopt, as well as the history of the adoption process, and with the initial encounter that was the foundation for the adoptive bond.

The challenge consists of going through adolescence like one goes through a health crisis rather than psychologically repeating the abandonment or rupture as it is experienced by the child in relation to his/her bond with his/her birth parents.

This mental health crisis should allow for a search for one's identity, based on the traces of one's origins, with the revival of transgenerational determinisms, by tying them in with those of his/her adopted lineage.

Deprived of a prevention which is, however, possible, adoptees are subject to an intensified kind of pressure that is tied in with the stigma of the filiation which targets them as "at risk", along with the intense awakening in the pubertal body of mnemonic traces of a buried drama, as well as with the ever-changing life forecast that is a distinctive feature of adolescence.

This pressure is presented through a symptomological inflation that comes about from a turning in on the self, or from utter dejection that results in suicidal ideation, and passes through diverse somatizations, addictive or delinquent behaviors, and even on through psychotic decompensation.

The transformation of the social bond, which leads to the removal of the protecting family, offers the adoptee a new opportunity to take stock of his/herself, to take over the responsibility for his/her future in spite of his/her young age, and to test reality in relation to the benefits of being resilient.

The common sequence becomes reversed and defines, in the passing, the "sound of mind, sound of body, fit for the street" logic for the psycho-bio-social health of adolescence.

The street reactualizes the ills of the soul and the body as well as the words of love and hope that preside over the separation from the biological parents and which lead to adoptive filiation.

6. REFERENCES

[1] A. REY, *Dictionnaire historique de la langue française* (A-L) Le Robert 1992 p23
[2] R Sandri, *Penser avec les bébés Ed Eres 1994* p63
[3] L Balestrière, *Freud et la question des origins* Ed De Boeck Université 1998 p235
[4] M-H Malandrin, *Le papa c'est celui qui dit, dans Lire Dolto aujourd'hui*, Ed Eres 2004 p24 –25
[5] F Juffer, *Adoptiekinderen, opvoeding en gehechtheid in het gezin* 1999
[6] Nazir Hamad *L'enfant adoptif et ses familles* Ed Denoël 2001
[7] D Drory C Frère *Le complexe de Moïse Regards croisés sur l'adoption* Ed Albin Michel 2006
[8] P. Kammerer, *Lire Dolto aujourd'hui: De la dette de vie à l'offre de parole en milieu éducatif* Ed Eres 2004 p95
[9] F Dolto, *Une éthique de la relation analytique* 1984 p141
[10] S. Sargueil *Maux d'Ados Un ouvrage pour comprendre votre corps quand il souffre, le soulager et le protéger* Ed De la Martinière Jeunesse 2003
[11] B. Graf Prof O. Halfon *Auto et hétéro agressivité à l'adolescence: entre suicide et homicide* Congrès Adolescence 1995 Bruxelles
[12] A. d'Alcantara Parentalité sociale et adoption homosexuelle *Revue Enfances Adolescence* N° 10/2006/1
[13] A. d'Alcantara *La santé mentale à l'école* Dans Au plus près des gens Ed FRB p182
[14] A. d'Alcantara Les poupées russes de l'adoption *Revue Enfances Adolescence* N° 8 2005/1
[15] A. d'Alcantara Ph van Meerbeeck *Adolescents: maturité physique, maturité psychique* Louvain Médical 2004 p5355-5357

In: The Adolescent Today in Medicine
Editors: N. Zdanowicz, et al. pp. 51-61
ISBN: 978-1-60021-764-7

Chapter 4

ATTACHMENT AND DEPRESSION IN ADOLESCENCE

Delvenne Véronique*

Psychiatrist, Free University of Brussels, Brussels

ABSTRACT

We must go to the obviousness that the nature of our early first relationships influence the whole course of our life just as well our personal relationships as the relation that we have with our health. It is during this first period of life that the child learns what he can await from humans relations and how he can react to stressful events. Theory of attachment researches in clinic populations has proposed a lot of interesting results about relation between quality of attachment and mental health mainly in child and adolescent population.

The experience of security is the goal of the attachment system, which is first and foremost a regulator of emotional experience. It lies at the heart of many forms of mental disorder. The attachment theory, developed by Bowlby, postulates that early experiences with the parents provide prototypes for all later relationships mediated by so called "internal working models".

At the time of adolescence, the transformation of the parental-child relationships imply an effort to become less dependent on care giving from primary attachment figures. It is also at this particular time that we can observe the impact of the quality of the first parental-child relationships as the adolescence is a time that reveals the quality of these first interactions and of the attachment type.

Increasing evidence indicates that high degree of insecure attachment is a predictor of subsequent severe depressive symptoms in adolescence. Evaluation of the quality of attachment style is also important in the psychotherapeutic project with the adolescent and his family.

So, to assure a good adolescent health, it is important to think about prevention at the early time of live and on the quality of mother-child interactions.

Keywords: adolescence, health, depression, attachment, family.

---

* Contact: Espace Thérapeutique Enfants-Adolescents-Parents, Rue Ketels 24, 1020 Bruxelles (Belgium) Tél : 0032497835076 Fax : : 003224611510, E.mail : v.delvenne@skynet.be

INTRODUCTION

Adolescence is defined as a time of great physical modifications, throughout the development of a sexual body. These tasks of adolescence request a lot of changes in interpersonal relationships such as a necessary distance with the parental figures. The influence of parents tends to lessen and peers become an increase source of support, values and sense of belonging. The autonomy in personal functioning increases progressively with modifications of social interactions and often complicated interpersonal relationships. In addition, adolescents faced with enormous changes in their formal operational thinking. They had to adapt to transitions to different schools. All these changes in the body, in interpersonal relationships and in social interests put a great strain to the Ego of the individual and are marked by increased stress. Mental health problems in adolescence are a combination of constitutional vulnerability, different life events and trauma experience, family environment, psychological and social factors but also difficulties in the attachment system.

EPIDEMIOLOGICAL HEALTH AND MENTAL HEALTH IN ADOLESCENCE

In a very large study on the adolescent health was made in France in 1988 [1]. M. Choquet and S. Ledoux have demonstrated that around 21 % of adolescent girls feel depressed (not a major depression) against 7 % of boys. In addition 33 % of these adolescents feel tired (boys 20 % and girls 35 %) and around 30 % had sleep difficulties mainly as falling asleep. In 1994 [2], the same authors have evaluated 14 278 youths between 11 and 19 years old, in general population with the Kandel scale for depression. 7.3 % of the adolescents had an elevated score of depression, 21.3 % a moderate score and 31.6 % a limit score with much more girls than boys who present depressive feelings. In addition, 23.4 % had suicidal ideas. Large reviews of the literature suggest that the prevalence of depressive disorders in the general adolescent population is between 4 and 8 % with 20 % of adolescents experiencing a diagnosable depressive episode by age 18 [3, 4]. In clinical populations, these estimates are much higher with a prevalence of 33 % of affective disorders at admission in a psychiatric unit [5].

The impact of dysthymia in the global health of the adolescents is major. Studies in school population of youth between 12 and 18 years old have showed that when they are in psychological suffering, the adolescents have much higher somatic complains such as headaches, gastric pain, nausea, back pain, tiredness… In addition, they consult much more frequently their family doctor or the school nurse for indistinct complains, depressive feelings, eating problems or sleep difficulties. These youth population is also much more exposed to suicidal acts [2, 6]. In addition, they showed certain continuity between sleep disturbance in infancy and addictive aptitude in adolescence.

Adolescence and Depression

The link between depressive feelings and alterations of global physical and mental health is very strong at the time of adolescence. In addition, sadness feeling is banal at that time of age with nearly 39 % of complain in the adolescent population [1]. A parental conflict, a disappointment in love, a bad result at school, leads the youth to a feeling of blues and moroseness. Generally, the teenager keeps a good reactivity with the external factors. He is still able to take pleasure if the opportunity arises. The culpability and the inhibition are non-existent. But it is essential to differentiate between a temporary feeling of sadness and a real depression of the adolescent. The major symptoms in the clinical picture of depressed adolescents are a greater alteration of the global health with a great sadness with negative thinking, less appetite, sleep disorders, inhibition and frequently anguish. School problems are frequent, sometimes until school dropouts or school refusal. The depreciation and a loss of self esteem are constant with a frequent withdrawal and a disinvestment from extra-school activities. Alcohol or drug abuse can occur frequently. The clinical picture is a little bit different following the sex. Girls are more likely to internalize their low mood with somatic complains whereas boys are more likely to behave on aggressive and delinquent manner with violence and acting out. In addition, depression often occurs in conjunction with other psychiatric disorders, such as conduct disorder or anxiety disorder [4, 7, and 8].

The consequences of adolescent depression can be devastating with a decrease in school performance, school drop-out, withdrawal from social relationships, and increase in family conflict, an increased risk of suicide but also an impact on global physical health. These factors also play a critical role in the maintenance and relapse of adolescent depression [7, 9].

From the Baby to the Adolescent: the Attachment Theory

We must go to the obviousness that the nature of our early first relationships influence the whole course of our life just as well our personal relationships as the relation that we have with our health. It is during this first period of life that the child learns what he can await from humans relations. The experience of security is the goal of the attachment system, which is first and foremost a regulator of emotional experience [10]. At the time of adolescence, we can observe the impact of the quality of the first parental-child relationships as the adolescence is a time that reveals the quality of these first interactions and of the attachment type.

Attachment theory postulates that early experiences with the parent provide prototypes for all later relationships mediated by so called «internal working models» [11, 12]. There is a universal human need to form close affectional bonds. Bowlby described attachment as a special type of social relationship, paradigmatically between infant and caregiver, involving an affective bond. More significantly, it may also be seen as the context within which the human infant learns to regulate emotion [13]. None of us is born with the capacity to regulate our own emotional reactions. A dyadic regulatory system evolves where the infant's signals of changes in state are understood and responded to by the caregiver, thereby becoming more regulated. The infant learns that arousal in the presence of the caregiver will not lead to disorganization beyond his coping capabilities. In states of uncontrollable arousal, the infant will come to seek physical closeness to the caregiver in the hope of soothing and the recovery of homeostasis. This model is described as the reflective function by Fonagy [14]. The stability of early childhood attachment patterns have been demonstrated, through the experience of the *Strange Situation* by Mary Ainsworth and her colleagues [15]. In this laboratory based procedure for observing infant's internal working models in action, infants of 18 months were briefly separated from their caregiver in a situation unfamiliar to them. They stay for some minutes with an unknown observer and than the mother come back. This procedure classifies infants and toddlers into one of four attachment categories various patterns of behavior. *Secure* infants explore readily in the presence of the primary caregiver, are distressed by their caregiver's departure and are anxious in the presence of the stranger. However, they rapidly seek contact with their mother when she come back following the brief period of separation, and are reassured by renewed contact. '*Anxious/Avoidant'* infants are usually made less anxious by separation, do not automatically seek proximity with the caregiver on her return following separation and may show no preference for the caregiver over the stranger. The '*Anxious/Resistant'* infant manifest impoverished exploration and play tend to be highly distressed by separation from the caregiver, but have great difficulty in settling after reunion, showing struggling, stiffness, or continued crying, or fuss in a passive way. The caregiver's presence or attempts at comforting fails to offer reassurance and their anxiety and anger appears to interfere with their attempts to derive comfort through proximity. A fourth group of infants are defined as '*Disorganised/ Disoriented*' while they appear to exhibit a range of seemingly undirected behavioral responses giving the impression of disorganization and disorientation [16]. These infants manifest freezing, handclapping, head banging and the wish to escape from the situation even in the presence of the mother. It is generally held that for such infants the caregiver has served both as a source of fear and as a source of reassurance, thus the arousal of the attachment behavioral system produces strong conflicting motivations. Not surprisingly, a history of severe neglect or physical or sexual abuse is often associated with the manifestation of this pattern [16]. Numerous empirical findings indicate that the development of a secure attachment with caregivers in the first years of life is related to higher sociability with other adults and children, higher compliance with parents and more effective emotional regulation [15]. Theory of attachment researches in clinical populations have proposed a lot of interesting results about relation between quality of attachment and mental health mainly in child and adolescent population [17]. It lies at the heart of many forms of mental disorder.

Attachment at the Time of Adolescence

Having a secure attachment in adolescence depends on different factors. First, the adolescent must have open communication with his parents. They had to be accessible and will provide him protection and help if he needed [15]. In that case, adolescent maintain a felt sense of security, a higher self esteem, much more positive peer relations and is able to develop greater autonomy seeking behavior [18-20].

At the time of adolescence, the transformation of attachment relationships implies an effort to become less dependent from primary attachment figures. The adolescent evolves from being a receiver of care from parents (including health care) to being a potential caregiver for a future infant. In addition, following changes in abstract reasoning abilities, adolescent begin to construct, from experiences with multiple caregivers, a more over arching stance toward attachment experiences [21]. Progressively, they view themselves as distinct persons differentiated from caregivers.

The parental role consists to give affection, to preserve a good health, to be available to children needs, to effectively negotiate the rules and the responsibilities and to pose clear limits. A deep and secure attachment will then be developed by the adolescent. This secure attachment with his/her parents is related to a healthy adaptation during adolescence and on the beginning of the adulthood, despite a reduction in adolescent and parent's interactions [22]. This teenager will be less likely to present problems of mental health and will be less inclined to consume drugs or to develop sexual risk behaviors [23-25]. In contrast, insecure attachment is met in situations with unavailability and unresponsiveness of the caregivers. These adolescent develop a negative schema of self and others and thus a vulnerability to depression. We should do more researches to determine the incidence of the major attachment on the cognitive style of the adolescent.

The quality of the adolescent relationships to peers is related to two main factors. First is the reciprocal emotional intimacy and self-disclosure. The second is the way in which parents represent their own relationships which were well evaluated by the Adult Attachment Interview [AAI, 21, 26]. In secure attachment style, adolescent manifest emotional openness and a capacity to reflect an emotional response and appropriately incorporate them into decisions and behaviors, including his self-care. Insecure adult style is expressed in terms of emotional avoidance, or increased emotional reactivity with negative emotions. Difficulties in life events are discussed and resolved within the family and thereby affect the child's own ability to generate mature solutions to various environmental problems.

So, secure and deep attachment during adolescence predisposes to better relationships to the parents and to the peers. Loneliness and the social rejection will be less present for these teenagers and they will adapt much more better to this social transition. They will present less signs of depression, anxiety or feelings of incompetence and have less aggressive or antisocial behaviors [27]. They have a better regard of themselves, have better strategies of adaptation enabling them to better react to the stress [23-27] and also a better general health. Attachment theorists have assumed that securely attached adults are more sensitive to their children's needs [28-29]. During periods of stress or danger or when they are in suffering, teenagers who are deeply attached to their parents, can lean on them and regard them as a home base from which they can reply new experiments. On the opposite, in same life difficulties, adolescents whose attachment with their parents is precarious or who had parents with little availability to their request, tend to avoid them and don't ask family support [18-19].

Attachment Insecurity and Depression in Adolescence

In 1980, Bowlby [12] suggested that some kinds of experiences in childhood are most likely to be associated to depression later in the lifetime. Separation from one's caregivers, mostly the mother, following death, or hospitalization can cause a sense of hopelessness and despair mostly if the child experiment little control over ensuing circumstances. Finally, this separation can be alarming to the global health as the infant will stop to eat and often to sleep until finally he can die. Secondly, when a child is unable to form a stable and secure relationship with the caregivers, he develops a model of the self as a failure. Finally, when a child experiment a relation with the parent in whom he received the message that he is incompetent or unlovable, he develops a model of the self as unlovable. Increasing evidence indicates that attachment insecurity is associated with vulnerability to depression in adolescence [30-32].

A very large, one year follow-up study was conducted in Norwee and have demonstrated that a high degree of insecure attachment is a predictor of subsequent severe depressive symptoms at follow-up among adolescents when controlled for depressive levels at the first time, various demographic and psychosocial factors and stress life events [31]. Another study has investigated security of parent and peer attachment among four groups of early adolescents: clinically depressed, nondepressed psychiatric controls, nonpsychiatric controls, and adolescents with resolved depression [30]. Depressed adolescents reported significantly less secure parent attachment than either of the control groups, and less secure peer attachment than the nonpsychiatric control group. Attachment security of adolescents with resolved depression was similar to that of the nonpsychiatric control group. Among all psychiatric patients, security of attachment to parents was negatively correlated with severity of depression. Less secure attachment to parents was also related to more maladaptive attribution styles, presence of separation anxiety disorder, and history of suicidal ideation.

In a group of adolescents who have been admitted in hospitalization for suicidal attempts, West [32] has found that adolescents who perceive their attachment figures as unavailable are overrepresented. They also have a high level of angry distress.

A number of models have been advanced to account for this association between attachment style and depression including emotion-regulation [33] and information-processing model [34]. Following the type of attachment, adolescent have different styles of affect regulation in social relationships with more distant and more hostile relations in the dismissing group and more anxiety and personal distress in the preoccupied group [33]. The role of interpersonal cognitions in the prediction of depression associated with interpersonal stressors had also been referred to the type of attachment, to the ability to be close to others and to anxiety about rejection and abandonment [34].

Representations of maternal figures as unavailable, unresponsive and unsupportive were significantly associated with high level of depression symptomatology in young adolescents [35]. However, these representations interact with stress in the prediction of depressive symptoms as attachment insecurity amplified the impact of interpersonal stress on depressive symptoms among adolescents [34, 36].

In populations of hospitalized adolescents in a crisis unit, for depressed problems, suicidal attempts, psychotic symptoms, we have observed [37] that the majority of them have had difficulties in the first time of life. Their internal insecurity but also their attachment style are mainly insecure or evitant. Means of defense which the teenager uses more readily, especially if its narcissistic bases are precarious are located in the register of omnipotence, megalomania and thus of refusal of assistance as well as acting out. The more the subject will be dependent on its internal objects the more request for assistance will be rejected violently.

Evaluation of Adolescent Mental Health and Propositions of Treatment

In first analysis, it is important to evaluate the request of care on an overall basis. Usually, adolescent does not have a personal request. He can not speak of him. He expresses his suffering by the language of the body. He is brought in the system of care at the request of an adult: school, parents, doctor, psychologist...

It is necessary to articulate the symptom on the context of the global health, with somatic, psychic, historical, relational and contextual dimensions suitable for the system and the individual. This task of evaluation imposes to the clinician, efforts of integration between various levels of comprehension in a continuous relationship between the somatic one, the psychic one and the interpersonal one.

At the time of first consultation, it is important to pay attention to the narrations, to the interactions between the patient and his parents but also to the nonverbal elements and somatic complains that are explain during the time of consultation and that often sign interpersonal defenses. A generation, the parent, carries the desire to consult, the adolescent is agreeing. With time, these positions evolve sometimes until being reversed. The various space times, individual and familial are alternated, according to the consultants and not in a pre-established order.

Within the framework of this global evaluation of health, various parameters will be taken into account to evaluate the type of therapeutic proposal that can be made. First, the age of the adolescent and his capacities of autonomy will be evaluated. Next, the therapist must appreciate the quality of the external reality, such as the quality of the relationships between the youth and his parents, the state of symbiosis or differentiation with them. Beginning an individual process without a sufficient differentiation with the family remains precarious and could be lived like destructor by the family. The environment of the adolescent including school, emotional relationships, relations to the peers, ... constitute important elements for evaluation of social support and social valorization. The evaluation of the mental adolescent functioning and also the quality of his physical health are essential. We have to evaluate the in-balance between objectal function and narcissism but also the types of defense mechanism and the potentialities of resistance to frustration.

When the symptoms and the suffering are distributed on the different members of the family with a low level of differentiation, it is an indication of family psychotherapy as first intervention. Taking into account, the interactive dimension of the symptom in a precondition is necessary to break in many cases, family alienation and to authorize in a second time the adolescent autonomy. Otherwise, there is a great risk of brutal interruption of the process, by a rigid family system which is opposed to any changes. When the group suffering is decreased, the family therapy can yield place to an individual psychotherapeutical work or a couple psychotherapy. At this stage of the evaluation, it is essential to be conscious that the choice and the strategy of interventions which could be installed depend on the adolescent and his parents and to what they can accept at that time of consultation but also of the epistemological characteristics of the therapist.

The first meetings with the adolescent prove to be capital. The quality of the adolescent's therapist needs tact, broadmindedness, flexibility and firmness but also authenticity to permit a true meeting. Confidence is not acquired at the beginning. It requires to be gained, to be consolidated. The psychotherapist offers himself like a new external object which can be used as a relay. He has to interest him to his internal world, to his history and to the origin of the conflicts subjacent of his symptoms. He has to allow the adolescent to create with him a potential space in which he can be in trust. This relation may allow the adolescent to view themselves as distinct from their caregivers and to experiment another attachment relationship with an adult different from his parent. We can speak about an identification meeting. The exits of the consultation will be multiple and to reinvent each time. It is often a step by step approach. The objective is then to support an evolutionary recovery.

Repairing attachment styles is an important way to propose treatment strategies. Following the hypothesis, within the relationship between depression and attachment style, some authors have developed some new way of treatment in the field of family therapy. Self evaluative and support seeking strategies could also represent targets for intervention [38]. Family need help to improve their communication skills, learn how to express positive feelings and learn about their adolescents' fear of abandonment and rejection. Attachment based therapy for families are interventions which focus on reconstructing secure attachment bounds [39]

CONCLUSION

So, to assure child and adolescent health, it is important to develop prevention in the early time of live mainly to preserve or to improve the quality of the mother-child interactions.

Theory of attachment researches in clinic populations have proposed a lot of interesting results about relations between the quality of attachment and the mental health mainly in child and adolescent populations. This quality of attachment is also important in the field of psychotherapeutic interventions with the adolescent and his family.

REFERENCES

[1] Choquet M., Ledoux S., Menke H. La santé des adolescents. La documentation Française. Ed INSERM, Paris 1988.

[2] Choquet M., Ledoux S. Adolescents – Enquête Nationale. Ed INSERM, Paris 1994.

[3] Birmaher B., Ryan N., Williamson D., Brent D., Kaufman J. Childhood and adolescent depression : a review of the past 10 years, part I. *J. Am. Acad. Child Adolesc. Psychiatry.* 1996; 35 (12): 1575-1583.

[4] Lewinsohn P.M., Hops H., Roberts R.E., Seeley J.R., Andrews J.A. Adolescent psychopathology: I. Prevalence and incidence of depression and other DSM III-R disorders in high school students. *J. of Abnorm. Psychol.* 1993; 102 (1): 133-144.

[5] U.S. Congress, Office of Technology Assistance. Adolescent health: vol 2. Background and the effectiveness of selected prevention and treatment services, OTA-H-466. Government printing office, Washington DC1991.

[6] De Clercq M., Vranckx A., Navarro F., Piette D. Enquête santé mentale des jeunes de l'enseignement secondaire en région de Bruxelles-capitale. Promes-ULB ed, Bruxelles 1996.

[7] Dunn V., Goodyer I.M. Longitudinal investigation into childhood- and adolescence-onset depression: psychiatric outcome in early adulthood. *Br. J. Psychiatry.* 2006; 188: 216-222.

[8] Lewinsohn P.M., Rohde P., Seeley J.R., Klein D.N., Gotlib I.H. Natural course of adolescent major depressive disorder in a community sample: predictors of recurrence in young adults. *Am. J. Psychiatry.* 2000; 157 (10): 1584-1591.

[9] Birmaher B., Brent D.A., Kolko D., Baugher M., Bridge J., Holder D., Iyengar S., Ulloa R.E. Clinical outcome after short-term psychotherapy for adolescents with major depressive disorder. *Arch. Gen. Psychiatry.* 2000; 57(1): 29-36.

[10] Sroufe l.A. Emotional development: The organization of emotional life in the early years. Cambridge University Press, New York, 1996.

[11] Bowlby I. Attachement et perte. Vol. 2: La séparation, angoisse et colère. PUF, Paris, 1973.

[12] Bowlby I. Attachement et perte. Vol 3: La perte. Tristesse et dépression. PUF, Paris, 1980.

[13] Sroufe L.A. An organizational perspective on the self. In D. Cicchetti and M. Beeghly (Eds), *The self in transition: Infancy to childhood.* (pp. 281-307). University of Chicago Press, Chicago, 1990.

[14] Fonagy P, Target M. Attachment and reflective function: their role in self-organization. *Dev. Psychopath.* 1997; 9 (4): 679-700.

[15] Ainsworth M.D.S., Blehar M.C., Waters E. and Wall S. Patterns of attachment: *A psychological study of the Strange Situation.* Hillsdale, NJ: Erlbaum, 1978.

[16] Main M., Solomon E. Procedures for identifying infants as disorganized/ disoriented during the Ainsworth Strange Situation. In D.C.M. Greenberg and E.M. Cummings (Eds), Attachment in the preschool years: Theory, research and intervention (pp. 121-160). University of Chicago Press, Chicago, 1990.

[17] Fonagy P., Steele M., Steele H., Leight T., Kennedy R., Mattoon G., Target M. Attachment, the reflective self, and bordeline states. In Goldberg S., Muir R., Kerr J. (Eds) *Attachment theory: social, developmental and clinical perspectives.* NJ: Analytic Press, Hilsdale, 1995: 233-278.

[18] Allen J.P., Hauser S.T. Autonomy and relatedness in adolescent-family interactions as predictors of young adults' states of mind regarding attachment. *Dev. Psychopath.* 1996; 8: 793-809.

[19] Allen J.P., Moore C., Kuperminc G., Bell K. Attachment and adolescent psychosocial functioning. *Child Dev.* 1998; 69 (5): 1406-1419.

[20] Allen J.P., Land D. Atttachment in adolescence. In J. Cassidy and P.R. Shaver (Eds). *Handbook of attachment: theory, research and clinical implications.* Guilford Press, New York, 1999: 319-335.

[21] Main M., Kaplan N., Cassidy J. Security in infancy, childhood and adulthood : a move to the level of representation. In Bretherton I., Waters E. (Eds) Growing points of attachment theory and research. *Monogr. Soc. Res. Child Dev.* 1985; 50 (1-2, n°209): 66-104.

[22] Ryan R.M., Deci E.L., Grolnick W.S. Autonomy, relatedness, and the self: Their relation to development and psychopathology. In D. Cicchetti and D. J. Cohen (Eds.), *Developmental psychopathology.* Vol. 1: Theory and methods. Wiley series on personality processes. Wiley, New York, 1995.

[23] Cooper M.L., Shaver P.R., Collins N.L. Attachment styles, emotion regulation, and adjustment in adolescence. *J. Pers. Soc. Psychol.* 1998; 74: 1380-1397.

[24] Jacobsen T., Edelstein W., Hofmann V. A longitudinal study of the relation between representations of attachment in childhood and cognitive functioning in childhood and adolescence. *Dev. Psychol.* 1994; 30 (1): 112-124.

[25] Kenny M. E., Donaldson G. A. Contributions of parental attachment and family structure to the social and psychological functioning of first-year college students. *J. Counsel Psychol.* 1991; 38 (4): 479-486.

[26] Main M., Goldwyn R. Adult attachment interview scoring and classification system. Unpublished manuscript, University of California at Berkeley, 1998.

[27] Papini, D.R., Roggman L. A. Adolescent Perceived Attachment to Parents in Relation to Competence, Depression, and Anxiety: A Longitudinal Study. *J. Early Adolesc.* 1992; 12: 420-440.

[28] Belsky J., Rosenberger K., Crnic C. The origins of attachment security: «Classical» and contextual determinants. In: S. Goldberg, R. Muir, J. Kerr (Eds.), *John Bowlby's attachment theory: historical clinical and social significance.* Analytic Press, Hillsdale, 1995: 153-184.

[29] De Wolff M.S., Van Ijzendoorn M.H. Sensitivity and attachment: a meta-analysis on parental antecedents of infant attachment. *Child Dev.* 1997; 68(4): 571-91.

[30] Armsden G.C., McCauley E., Greenberg M.T., Burke P.M., Mitchell J.R. Parent and peer attachment in early adolescent depression. *J. Abnorm. Child Psychol.* 1990; 18(6): 683-97.

[31] Sund A.M., Wichstrom L. Insecure attachment as a risk factor for future depressive symptoms in early adolescence. *J. Am. Acad. Child Adolesc. Psychiatry.* 2002; 41(12): 1478-85.

[32] West M.L., Spreng S.W., Rose S.M., Adam K.S. Relationship between attachment-felt security and history of suicidal behaviours in clinical adolescents. *Can. J. Psychiatry.* 1999; 44(6): 578-82.

[33] Koback R.R., Sceery A. Attachment in late adolescence: working models, affect regulation, and representations of self and others. *Child Dev.* 1988; 59(1): 135-46.

[34] Hammen C.L., Burge D., Daley S.E., Davila J., Paley B., Rudolph K.D. Interpersonal attachment cognitions and prediction of symptomatic responses to interpersonal stress. *J. Abnorm. Psychol.* 1995; 104(3): 436-43.

[35] Shirk S.R., Gudmundsen G.R., Burwell R.A. Links among attachment-related cognitions and adolescent depressive symptoms. *J. Clin. Child Adolesc. Psychol.* 2005; 34(1): 172-81.

[36] Murray L., Halligan S.I., Adams G., Patterson P., Goodyer I.M. Socioemotional development in adolescents at risk for depression: the role of maternal depression and attachment style. *Dev. Psychopathol.* 2006; 18(2): 489-516.

[37] Delvenne V., Debry M., Janssens N. Nicolis H., Geuzaine C. Adolescents in crisis : structural lines, symptoms and quality of attachment. Presented at the 5th congress of

the International Society for Adolescent Psychiatry. Aix-en-Provence, 1999, abstract book p 10.

[38] Diamond G., Siqueland L. Diamond G.M. Attachment-based family therapy for depressed adolescents: programmatic treatment development. *Clin. Child Fam. Psychol. Rev.* 2003; 6(2): 107-27.

[39] Herring M., Kaslow N.J. Depression and attachment in families: a child-focused perspective. *Fam. Process.* 2002; 41(3): 494-518.

In: The Adolescent Today in Medicine
Editors: N. Zdanowicz, et al. pp. 63-68
ISBN: 978-1-60021-764-7

Chapter 5

CRISIS INTERVENTION MODEL WITH ADOLESCENT PRESENTING SOMATIC COMPLAINTS IN EMERGENCY PSYCHIATRY

Vincent M. Dubois*
Psychiatrist, Head of psychiatric service,
Cliniques universitaires St-Luc, Université Catholique de Louvain, Belgium

ABSTRACT

The crisis intervention with adolescents is first a dynamic approach that distances itself from any attempt to reduce all adolescent's psychiatric illness to the crisis or to consider the crisis as a new illness. Different authors differentiate between the notion of crisis and that of illness within an overall framework incorporating the patients and their families, the psychiatric institutions, and the social systems. In this context, the crisis represents an element that evolves in discontinuity and that is produced by the illness itself or is upstream of the illness, wich, in contrast is static and is, as it were, suspended in a period of crisis. Homeostasis is therefore interrupted during this period of discontinuity, an event that may result in destructuring or, alternatively, restructuring on the basis of some newly established balance. The crisis lends a more normal and everyday image to adolescent's suffering and provides a more dynamic interpretation of the therapeutic aims. When a health crisis occurs with adolescents, the patient or, more frequently, the patient's family turn to emergency department in search of immediate help. In this context, crisis intervention is able to offer an interesting mode of response to adolescent's crisis, especially when presenting somatic complaints.

Keywords: adolescent health, crisis intervention, emergency psychiatry.

---

* Contact: Clinique St Luc, avenue E. Mounier, 1200 Bruxelles (Belgium) Tél : 003227641111 Fax : : 003227642075, E.mail : dubois@pscl.ucl.ac.be

1. Increase of Cases of Teenagers Psychiatric Emergencies

Since a few years, several authors revealed that the number of adolescents presenting to the Emergency Department (ED) with psychiatric emergencies is increasing a lot [1-3]; especially in the cities, where the incidence of psychiatric cases among teenagers is strikingly growing.

According to the World Health Organization (WHO), childhood neuropsychiatric disorders will become one of the five most common causes of morbidity, mortality and disability for adolescents all around the world by the year 2020 [4].

The main symptoms leading to a visit to the ED are, among other things, suicidal behaviors, acts of self destruction, sexual abuse or violence, alcoholism, drug addiction, delusions, agitation, panic attacks and somatoform disorders. According to De Clercq and Cassiers [5], in approximately 70 % of these cases, the symptoms presented reflect a family or individual crisis situation.

An explanation to such an increase in adolescent psychiatric emergencies can be given by several socio-cultural factors, among which the demise of the extended family, the rise of feeble single-parent cells, the degradation of social links and the proliferation of violence in the urban regions.

Given this book's subject on adolescent's health and the number of somatoform disorders in teenagers presenting to ED, this chapter is not meant to be a full study of all the adolescent psychiatry acute symptomatology and its management. Instead, we will try and develop a crisis intervention model suitable with different types of somatic complaints.

2. The Main Features of Emergency Psychiatry

2.1. The Crisis Mechanisms

The crisis is generally due to a deep break in the patient's mental functioning and also in the family context, as an answer to important changes or existential problems that must be confronted [6]. The crisis, characterized by somatic or mental symptoms, is then generated because neither the patient nor his family can solve the problem.

The symptoms then keep growing and, once they become intolerable for the patient and his environment, they require urgent help. The emergency can therefore be compared to the visible part of an iceberg. In such emergency situations, the patient and the family often go for help at the ED of a general hospital, which they find suitable because of its accessibility.

2.2. Importance of Somatic Complaints

During adolescence, the somatoform disorders most likely to occur and require a visit to the ED is conversion disorder [3]. At first, most teenagers consult an internal medicine specialist, a surgeon or a pediatrician about their physical disorder, as a last chance call to doctors to help him and stop the crisis.

2.3. The Families Are to Be Involved

In order to help the patient, it is generally necessary to establish a working alliance [7] with him and his family. Therefore, it is very important to let both sides express themselves and evaluate the importance of what they feel in their daily context.

3. Interventions Objectives when Dealing with Teenagers with Somatic Complaints

3.1. The Therapeutic Triangulation

Mostly, adolescents going through psychological or psychiatric problems go to the ED only with a somatic complaint [8] and generally ask to see a doctor and no psychiatrist. If there is no triangulation and the psychiatrist sees the patient directly on request of the internist who is convinced that the problem etiology is psychiatric, the following care program is often bound to fail:

[1] The patient has the feeling that he has been abandoned by the somatician in the hands of the psychiatrist he had not even asked for. In most cases, no somatic investigation has been carried out.
[2] The patient could become aggressive towards the psychiatrist just because he does not understand the change from the medical to the psychological approach.
[3] The psychiatrist often finds himself in an awkward position because of the surgeon request, who explained his intervention too few, too bad or not at all.
[4] Last thing – which might be the most important problem – the situation between the psychiatrist and the patient is reversed and the psychiatrist has to convince the patient that he needs help.

Therefore, when dealing with somatoform disorders or suspected suicidal attempts in teenagers, the internist systematically calls out the psychiatrist for a “triangular therapeutic triangulation interview”.

Thus, when every organic etiology has been discarded and the internist is persuaded that the patient is suffering from a psychiatric problem, he then calls a psychiatrist to arrange an interview between the patient, the internist and the psychiatrist. Whenever possible, the familiars should be invited to the triangulation interview.

The planning and achieving of the triangulation interview are essential to the good establishing and follow-up of the care program. At first, the internist has to explain the patient’s reasons for coming to the ED, the examinations that have been realized, the first diagnosis hypotheses, the results and why hospitalization or a somatic treatment are of no use. Then, the patient, his family and even the psychiatrist can ask questions to the internist.

In the second phase, the internist has to tell the patient that he has a true problem of anxiety or depression, even though the examination results are negative and that the patient will not be sent right back home after having been told that “There’s nothing wrong with you”. The internist then explains that the patient’s problem is within the scope of expertise of one of his colleagues, which was present during the triangulation interview and which is the psychiatrist. This way, the psychiatrist's intervention is not felt by the patient as a punishment and there is no "abandon feeling" from his part either.

At the third step, the psychiatrist can question the patient about the internist's point of view. The psychiatrist can thus get an idea of what representations the patient has of his trouble and his personal and family history towards psychiatry. Little by little, the psychiatrist aims to build a therapeutic alliance between him and the patient [9], which is often a key to success.

In most cases, the patient will be alone during the interview with the psychiatrist once the internist position is clearly defined and the patient knows when he can contact him again. Half the time, family members will assist to the interview or will be involved later on.

3.2. Analysis of the Crisis' Whole System

Some fundamental questions should be asked when in front of acute crisis symptoms: "What is at the origin of the emergency? Who is suffering from a crisis? What is the real meaning of this call for help?" Often, the patient and his family are confirmed that they can not continue to cope with the patient's problem by the direct intervention of the emergency psychiatry team, which decides to hospitalize the patient or to give him medication.

3.3. Negotiation of a Therapeutic Alliance with a Teenager and His Family

As already said, the most important thing during the first moments is the establishing of a therapeutic alliance instead of the evaluation, diagnosis or treatment decision. The therapeutic alliance is a sort of tacit contract between the patient, who is experiencing an acute crisis, and the therapeutic team.

The therapeutic team must then use intervention techniques which goal is to create the therapeutic alliance.

4. Crisis Intervention

4.1. The Suggestion of an Intensive Care Program

Generally, patients and their family go to a general hospital ER because they think it the right place to get helped during day or night when they feel the situation has become unendurable.

A few things have to be explained to the patient and his family when dealing with them at the ED:

1. That the gravity of the patient's situation is taken into account.
2. That we are aware of the family's distress and pain.

3. That they were right to come to ER and that it was the good decision to make because their situation is serious and something has to be done immediately.
4. That the care already received by the patient was good but not enough or that something new blew it all up.
5. That we can help them by setting up an intensive care program.
6. That they will be taken care of during the course of the intensive care program by the same persons they have just met.
7. That the family and the GP have to collaborate in order to get to a solution.

4.2. Crisis interaction

This is the first part of the intensive care program and it can go on from one to two weeks. The two objectives that are to be pursued are as follows:

1. During the first interviews, a therapeutic alliance has to be built with the family and the patient, and it should be further developed to turn it into a genuine working alliance [9].
2. Rather than focusing on the patient's symptoms, the first thing to do is pinpoint the crisis hypotheses that are probably at the origin of the urgent request.

This phase of crisis interaction is one of great research and thinking for the caregivers' team as all the dimensions of the patient's situation are considered and analyzed.

All this research work helps the crisis team to formulate one or several crisis hypotheses. Consequently, the patient's problems, which at first were only somatic, change to a more circular logic deep in their family and their own mind.

At the end of this phase, the change from an "external" to an "internal" register allows the caregivers, the patient and the family to express the problem which is to be dealt with during the following step, which is the intervention phase.

4.3. Crisis Intervention

This phase, as opposed to the previous one, will concentrate on the patient's problem and not any more on the examination of the patient's every dimension. The crisis intervention phase may last up to three months and is generally carried out by one or two specific therapists.

This phase's goal has to be described and discussed with the patient and his family at the end of the previous one.

In such adolescent crisis situations, a "separate" approach is the only way to respect the need to speak and suffering of both generations; because if we focus on the teenager's individual follow-up, we are exposed to the family opposition and on the other side, if we establish a systemic family approach with both the teenager and the family, the adolescent will generally go back into his shell, which makes it complicated for the counselor to mobilize the situation.

Therefore, the psychiatrist (or psychologist) who reached the best therapeutic alliance with the teenager receives the charge of the individual follow-up and the other therapist will go on with the family. This plan has to be suggested and explained to both sides at the end of the interaction phase. The family and the adolescent also have to be told that during the interviews, every secret that is presented as such will be respected by both counselors. From time to time, combined interviews are planned with the teenager, his parents and both therapists in order to evaluate the evolution of the intergenerational communication .

4.4. Negotiation of the Follow-Up

At the end of the intervention phase (generally after three months), we plan a last interview with the teenager, the family, their therapists and a therapist from the Community Mental Health Services to suggest a follow-up after the crisis intervention, because this follow-up is impossible to realize with the ED staff. It is therefore very important to develop cooperation links with the Community Mental Health Services outpatient psychiatry network.

Nevertheless, these collaboration attempts are quite difficult to organize, because the general hospital is frequently inward-looking and manages the situations as if it were the only structure able to do it, but also because the outpatient network is not much involved in dealing with psychiatric emergencies coming from the general hospital.

These are the reasons why particular working relations between general hospital and ambulatory structures must absolutely be increased.

REFERENCES

[1] Page D. Pediatric psychiatry : more blues in ED? *Hosp. Health Netw.* 2000; 74:24.

[2] Haugh R. A crisis in adolescent psychiatry. *Hosp. Health Netw.* 2003; 77:12.

[3] Edelsohn GA, Gomez JP. Psychiatric emergencies in adolescents. *Adolesc. Med.* 2006; 17 : 183-204.

[4] Ringeisen H, oliver KA, Menvielle E. Recognition and treatment of mental disorders in children : considerations for pediatric health systems. *Pediatr. Drugs.* 2002; 4:697-703.

[5] DeClercq M, Cassiers L. Crisis intervention in the face of emergencies; *Acta psychiatrica Belgica.* 1990; 90:81-99.

[6] DeClercq M, Dubois V. Crisis intervention models in the French-speaking countries. *Crisis.* 2001; 22; 201-208.

[7] Andreoli A. Working alliance as a predictor of crisis intervention long-term outcome. In *Psychiatry : A world perspective.* Elsevier, Amsterdam, 1990.

[8] DeClercq M. The therapeutic triangle : an essential tool in dealing with crisis. *JEUR.* 1990; 3 : 107-112.

[9] Andreoli A, Lalive J, Garrone G. Crisis and crisis intervention in psychiatry. *SIMEP,* Paris, 1986.

In: The Adolescent Today in Medicine
Editors: N. Zdanowicz, et al. pp. 69-88
ISBN: 978-1-60021-764-7

Chapter 6

PATIENTS HAVE FAMILIES

Christine Reynaert*
Psychiatrist, Head of psychiatric service, Cliniques universitaires
Mont-Godinne, Université Catholique de Louvain

« The idea that the individual can be analized as separate from the system of relationships of which he or she forms an integral part is the fundamental epistemological error of western thought»
M. Selvini-Palazzoli (1974) [1]

« Your ultimate capacity to be an autonomous, self-sufficient person is directly linked to your capacity to be a part of and to really belong to others »

C. Whitaker (1998) [2]

ABSTRACT

In spite of the frantic individualism extolled by our societies, we are all interacting individuals. The significant relationships that we nurture with our relatives influence them and are influenced by them. This interactive and systemic approach can apply to any issue and age in life since the presence of suffering in one individual sparks emotional reactions among family members, and necessitates the development of their adaptive skills. This approach in relational dynamics is particularly appropriate with respect to adolescent problems. Adolescence is indeed an intermediate period of life in between self-actualization and autonomy. Many difficulties and health-related disorders are caused in part by adolescents' individual psychosomatic economy, but also by the difficulties parental figures encounter as they try to reorient themselves toward a new lifecycle. Parents find themselves facing each other and confronting couple difficulties that may have been concealed during the years that were devoted to child rearing. Behind a façade of rebellious opposition, many adolescents are in reality extremely sensitive and

* Contact: Clinique Mont-Godinne, avenue E. Thérasse, 5530 Yvoir (Belgium) Tél : 003281423751 Fax : 003281423753, E.mail : christine.reynaert@psme.ucl.ac.be

preoccupied by their family's and parental couple's future. Helping them confront their own self-interrogations will often involve unmasking family difficulties and helping the parental couple restart an active restructuring of their dyad.

The present chapter reviews the major authors who have examined the difficulties that certain families experience when adapting to changes that are imposed by adolescence. In particular, Minuchin, Stierling, and Mara Selvini have described the characteristics of such families: rigid, hyper-protective, entangled, and avoiding conflict resolution.

These authors' theories will be illustrated with clinical examples which show how intervening both simultaneously and parallel with the family network and with the adolescent patient increases therapeutic efficiency.

Keywords: adolescence, families, interactions.

1. Towards a Systems Approach

Calling to mind a patient's family and circle immediately reminds one that in a materialistic technological society in which individualism is extolled, the true meaning of life is to be found in emotional intimacy and the warmth of emotional bonds.

It is unfortunate that medicine does not integrate this dimension for a bio-psychosocial approach.

The family transmits from one generation to the next genetic and psychological baggage, behaviors based on myths, certain beliefs, and some secrets, but also some glory and shameful incidents from the past. Furthermore, the family constitutes a scenario where it isn't that easy to form strong emotional bonds and remain attached to one another while each is developing his/her freedom, creativity, and the feeling of being the author of his/her life, and for our purpose, of his/her health and quality of life.

It is inside of the family that we experience alternating states of dependence and autonomy, an oscillating that we readjust within each relational context with the diverse members of our immediate circle.

Human beings have a reciprocal influence on one another. Our self-awareness depends on our significant others but we can also have an influence on them.

The family systems therapy approach focuses on these reciprocal relational interactions. A family constitutes a group, although certainly a small one, but also an interactional system. It would therefore be important for every doctor to pay attention to evaluating the psychological states of the individuals in his/her group of patients, but also to the type of interactions that are formed between them and others in their case and the place of the illness in all of that. Does the illness originate from a rapprochement, a distancing, a game of fools, or conflicted communication?

Generally, family systems writers are in agreement when they say that the family is a whole unit and when an illness affects one of its members, the other members are also affected by the situation and they have to call on their adaptive mechanisms, to a very high degree.

These required changes represent a crisis situation for the family. This crisis occasions an upset in the usual equilibrium. The family is going to have to reorganize itself to correct this imbalance and restore a certain amount of homeostasis.

What is more, the family systems approach is not a therapy on the skewer of the diverse psychotherapies in existence. Its theoretical corpus introduces a fundamental epistemological rupture, another reading of the approach: a symptom is no longer only considered a characteristic of an individual but also the product of the interactions between the members of the system. The system which the therapist is the most invested in and which is the most accessible to him/her is, in general, that of the family.

Nevertheless, the concepts and intervention strategies which family systems psychotherapy resorts to (circularity of communication, alliance with the system, researching of the function of the system, and positive refocusing) can be applied to other networks or systems (the community).

The title of our chapter is also that of one in Richardson's book. He is an inspired generalist and a fine observer who already in 1948 [3] noted that families exist in which there is always at least more member who is bearing the burden of a symptom. When one member of the family is cured, another falls ill. According to him, these families seem particularly confused, with little expression of aggressivity and an apparent need to always be in a relationship with medical personnel.

Our own work [4] corroborated the relationship of expressed aggressivity in relating with the occurrence of psychosomatic pathologies. These observations are in accord with the idea that the non-expression of emotions remains the tell-tale sign of psychosomatic illness and with the psychoanalytic description of the subject at risk for contracting psychosomatic ailments. The concepts of alexithymia and operational thinking come to mind.

If taking into account the quality of social support (neither rejecting nor hyperprotective) must be a part of the art of healing for every patient, this necessity appears to be even more obvious in the case of an adolescent who is presenting with health problems.

2. Adolescents Have Families

For a long time now, in our societies, adolescence has no longer been considered just the biological phenomenon of puberty. On the contrary, it now designates the passage from childhood to adulthood, a passage that extends over several years (from pre-adolescence through young adulthood) and is therefore a true lifecycle. It has to do rather with the most stressful period of life for an individual. The formation of sexual identity reawakens infantile traumas and non-resolved Oedipal difficulties. Moreover, it is at the time of adolescence that the majority of mental illnesses break forth (schizophrenia, anorexia, and other confusions which can be expressed through anxious/depressive and/or somatic disorders). Adolescent specialists have elaborated explanatory models about this period of psychological fragility, models which are essentially centered on the individual.

If a health problem arises with a young person, one generally approaches it from the classical medical point of view. In cases where there is a linear somatic progression and what science can offer seems insufficient, one then turns towards the modern, sophisticated concept of individual destiny, namely the unconscious as it is defined by psychoanalysis.

From the somatic point of view, the adolescent body makes a lot of noise. The creation of a feeling of wholeness depends on the psychosomatic integration of this bodily maturation process. There is corporeal self with internal and exterior boundaries. It is very important that during the course of these identity development stages that the child who has become an adolescent has the feeling that he/she is inhabiting his/her own body. Obviously, a sustaining attitude that is neither trivializing nor dramatizing is to be expected from the adult.

Like during the mirroring stage of young childhood, the consolidation of narcissism allows the adolescent to no longer be held back within his/her body and within the world of childhood. The operation is all the more successful when the parents' regard for the child brings about positive and sustaining feelings. One's self-image can then be whole, sexual, and have boundaries.

The representation of the body acquires its role from the traces of the parents desire to have a child which is what sustains one's identity and initiation into sexuation. And this shows up like a plus, the producer of young adults' future history [5, 6].

For the girl, puberty is marked by the arrival of the menses. Pleasure in this is not automatic and female sexuality makes it debut, one will understand, in a more diffuse way that is tied in with the emotions of love, a fact that doesn't mean that the latter will be less intense [7]. What the mother says about this has a lot of importance for the adolescent girl. She might say, "My poor girl, every month, from now on, you're going to suffer like me and like my mother did before me. We both suffered though it," Or conversely, "Angel-there's another woman in the house now." The young girl will exhibit seductive behaviors toward her father who, if he marvels at her in a way that is healthy and makes her feel secure, will give her confidence in herself.

The boy, from the sole fact of high hormone levels, will come to know sexual excitation and orgasm at the time of puberty. Very quickly, he will recognize that his penis is the primary source of his pleasure and he will repeat, compelled by his sexual urge, this new and intense pleasure that he discovered.

We understand that men think they can gratify their narcissistic psychoaffective needs and their need to have fusion through sexuality. The man's point of fragility will be on the level of sexual performance. All analysts will say that the place of the father is very important at this time of life. The boy must identify with the masculine values of the paternal image.

Adolescence is also, and above all else, a psychological concept [8]. The child who has more or less succeeded in his/her journey has constructed a personal identity in the sense that he/she has been able to maintain security within. He/she is confronted by successive stages of privation and frustrations, something that is expressed through internal and external conflicts.

At the end of childhood, the adolescent must mourn for the way he/she has lived, for what caused him/her to live, and for what he/she used to love. This mourning imposes a stage in which the question of why and how to live turns up. "What is the meaning of life? What is it that is good for me and what is not? What are my limits and those of others?"

This stage is marked by the disappearance of all the childhood objects of interest up until the time one becomes an adult. One will decide on a series of other interests with a series of goals. But between the two stages there is an emptiness, an emptiness that generally causes the adolescent to suffer because he/she doesn't know who he/she wants to be. All that he/she knows is that he/she doesn't want to be the child that he/she has been.

Into this emptiness that adolescents experience, and which makes depression a relatively normal phase, the question of death may enter.

For want of feeling alive, symbolizing, and being able to fantasize about an actual and future family romance, he/she runs the risk of positioning him/herself in dangerous situations that will cause him/her to experience some things through certain emotions that will be produced.

Young people for whom there is no longer any interior world, where there is no longer a trace of anything, are always making attempts at self-determination, but without words, only through actions or objects (brand-name school bags, the latest cell phones or MP3's). [9]

Growing bigger necessitates a certain amount of violent behavior that, when it is mediatized by language, turns into aggressivity. Aggressivity is structural with adolescents and allows them to fight with their parents in order to win emancipation, to affirm themselves, to defend a certain number of values, but above all, so that they can prompt a diminution of the parents' power over themselves. This change is not just to be understood as adolescent development of the self but also as a step whereby he/she takes over part of the responsibility for him/herself that his parents formerly had.

One can observe this situation in the domain of health. If in childhood it is the parents who decide when one is going to the doctors, when one takes medicine, etc., when the adolescent advances in age, he/she takes over this power [10].

We do indeed see that remarks from parents like, "Don't forget to brush your teeth," "Put on some heavy clothes; you're going to catch cold," are protective behaviors from one's childhood that are no longer acceptable during adolescence. This struggle to take over control of one's health is made very difficult if the adolescent has difficulties symbolizing and verbalizing the impulses than run through him/her.

Our families don't make this step easy. Indeed, an egalitarian ideal of democracy reigns in this area and the place of the child is, without a doubt, too central, as much in united families as in families where the parents have divorced and in which a hyper-preoccupation with the child's well being prevails and makes it impossible to say "no" to him/her and impose some authority. Because of this lack of limits, the child's capacities for mentalization are not called upon. The child no longer benefits from the smallest of privations that would allow him/her to formulate plans, experience an imaginary world, and project him/herself into the future. Therefore, one recommends that parents assume an attitude of negotiation, of renouncing some actions of authority. Laxity and excessive tolerance is often interpreted by the adolescent as indifference. One therefore asks parents to intelligently and creatively yield a portion of their power. [11]

One asks a lot of parents then if they are capable of so much flexibility! It is at this point that a family systems approach can enlighten and supplement the resource of medical and psychiatric personnel who take responsibility for adolescent health problems. Too often, one considers the parents to be supportive assets who are touchy about giving us details of their heteroanamnesis, and not often enough, as co-therapists who could help us in our taking charge. We should particularly consider them as persons who are also suffering, who need to be sustained, and who are deserving of all our empathetic attention and care.

3. A Phase of the Lifecycle…For the Whole Family

The complex process of maturation, and all its foreseeable complications in the domain of physical and mental health, does not just have to do with the adolescent. It is important to contextualize it in the intergenerational report in which the new generation is recognized by the generation that is actually “in command.” The symbolic order of the succession of generations requires the inscription of the subject into his/her generation and the symbolic line of demarcation that allows not only membership with, but difference between the generations.

This definition sets forth the intergenerational bond that constitutes a family’s history. It does not concentrate the weight of the “adolescent phenomenon” on the shoulders of its young actors but the weight of the issues is resolutely distributed along the top of the preceding generations. What place in life do the adult parents and mature grandparents leave for young people? And are these older generations ready to hand over the torch to the adolescent and recognize to the place that he/she is to occupy?

The adolescent thus summons the preceding generations for the losses specific to each life phase, but perhaps also specific to the starting up of other pleasures.

Leaving one’s place behind is not an easy step to take, above all in a society like ours where the prevailing culture is all “adolescentric” and where looking young is the model for the entire society! [8]. The concept of the family lifecycle [9] has allowed for the clarification of the problems of separation at the time of adolescence. Thus, the transgenerational rules of different family systems of origin are found to be reactualized by children’s impulse to be autonomous. Adolescent difficulties start to resonate as their grandparents enter into the last phase of their lives. There is the reconfrontation in the case of the parents, on the one hand because of their own dynamics as a couple, and on the other hand, on account of a double separation, ie., the separation from their child (the empty nest syndrome), and often at the same time, because of a mourning process for their own parents who can fall ill or die during this period of the life cycle.

If the parental couple has known how to maintain a zone of complicity, trust, and intimacy, they will have no difficulty in rediscovering themselves as a couple and reinvesting in their emotional and sexual intimacy. Furthermore, if each individual in the couple has succeeded in maintaining a flexible swinging back and forth between autonomy and dependence, they will not have any difficulties reinvesting themselves in intellectual, artistic, or sports activities that they didn’t have the time to develop while the children were young.

If the equation that constitutes a couple is rather complex in the opening/closing up of movement in their relationship, the equation created by a couple involved in parenting proves to be even more complex since it is confronted by the mysterious ascent inherent with the appearance of a third person: the child.

For the child triangulates the couple, but in a way that is so distinctive that everything unfolds without it seeming to be a true triangulation. Initially included in the couple’s “we,” the adolescent has to detach him/herself to create his/her own “I.”

In fact, with a lot of couples nowadays, the triangulation that the state of being parents generates also becomes, little by little, a triangulation when the “we” of the parental couple has been absorbed by the children with possible regression in relation to the risks of emotional investments. Therefore, there is a risk that the children will act as strangers at a later time when they themselves are confronted by an intimacy with the parents that is often difficult to reassume. [12]

If the child, as a third person, has acted as a camouflage for the underlying marital conflicts, one can understand how he/she will have a difficult time leaving his/her parents to battle with problems that they never resolved or even approached!

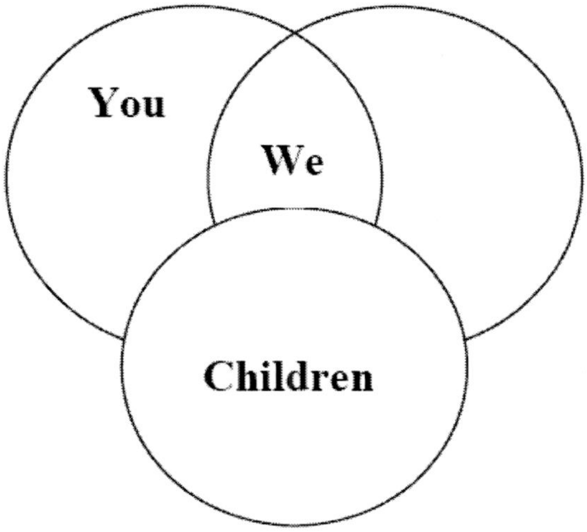

A lot of family therapists hold the conviction that it is the children who are the great healers of the parents' hidden wounds. This concept is utilized above all in clinical practice as a strategy for diverting the family's attention away from the adolescent's escapades. The adolescent finds him/herself very surprised and relieved when he/she learns that his/her parents had problems themselves when they were adolescents or that they are experiencing problems as a couple. Then, he/she isn't the only one who has problems!

It is rather distressing for some parents who haven't realized all their aspirations to discover themselves faced with young, seductive individuals outside of themselves who have plenty of plans for their own lives. One will note that a good number of extra-marital relationships and couple breakups are concomitant with their children's adolescence. Clinical observations completely demonstrate the importance of the repercussions of the process of separation on family dynamics.

Stierlin, 1981 [13], describes three separation modalities:

1. In the first illustrative case, the adolescent maintains a very close bond within the family circle. The parents, like the adolescent, reveal themselves to be incapable of redefining their relationships on new bases. They are not ready to confront sufferings that are comparable to those that mourning, on account of separation, provokes.
2. In other cases, the separation is forgotten about, based on the rejection mode. The adolescent is devalued and expelled from the family unit; these brutal ruptures come about more frequently in families that have broken up.
3. The third mode is that of delegation. Adolescents benefit from a limited step towards autonomy but they must accomplish tacit missions that often overwhelm them. For example, one adolescent has to satisfy family expectations as regards social success while another will have as his/her mission to attack one parent on the part of the other. These delegations are seen in families where the couples are together, as well as in single-parent families.

Therefore, when a health problem becomes chronic with a young person and we are looking for factors of stress, one mustn't buy an explanation outside of the family too quickly (school difficulties, a disappointment in love, etc). But rather, we should completely broaden our perspective regarding the family system and proceed to an analysis of the function of the symptom. During the time that the young person has experienced problems, have the parents understood one another better, not as well, or about the same? Have the family members been talking more inside of the family?

This fact emphasizes that the parents could probably be the object of our attention as doctors. We should not hesitate to call upon the family systems as a whole more often when dysfunction appears inside of the family organization.

Examples:

1. If a mother seems over-invested in relation to the care she gives to her sick child, it is easy to bring into the medical consultation a short sentence such as, "That's great-it's extraordinary how courageous of a mother you are. But don't you ask the child's father for any help?"
2. If we see a couple who doesn't seem to know how to talk about anything besides their worries about their children, we shouldn't hesitate to advise them to go out by themselves once a week and do activities as a couple again.

4. Theoretical Points of Reference

For G. Bateson [14], the bonds between the members of a group are situated at the level of communication. All communication implies a speaker who transmits a message, to a recipient. But in return, the recipient happens to have an influence on the speaker? Properly speaking then, it has to do with an interaction. Bateson's analysis of communication styles is based on the discoveries of the Palo Alto school. Watzlawich has summarized the foremost axioms regarding communication in his famous work entitled Pragmatics of Human Communication [15]:

1. It is impossible not to communicate.
2. Every communication introduces two aspects: the content of and rules for a relationship (one will understand that parent/child rules change at adolescence).
3. The nature of a relationship is to be reconfigured in a circular form by the sequence of communication between two partners (redundant or creative interactions): we review repetitious parent/child disputes, without a resolution of these conflicts.
4. All exchange of communication is symmetrical or complementary (adolescence entails a diminution of complementarity, to the advantage of symmetry).
5. Human beings use two modes of communication: digital and analog (verbal and non-verbal language), that is, movements and expressions of the body and tone of voice. One knows only too well just how often the adolescent can send us double messages when these two languages are not congruent.

The most obvious example of this is the anorexic mental patient who is thin and skeleton-like and who says that, "Everything's alright except that I think I'm a little too fat!"

With this model we leave behind one that is only based on the transformation of individual energies for one that invests in the creation and transmission of information. Therefore, when a problem occurs, it is the result of misunderstandings in communication. This model has important implications for practice. Interesting ourselves in the communication between a young person and his/her parents helps us to remain neutral and careful, so as to not take sides.

Credit goes back to Helm Stierlin [16] for having described the peculiarities of "counter-transference" in family treatment that involves adolescents. The multiplicity of levels on which conflicts of mission and loyalty are situated often throws therapy off track or causes a risk that the therapist might give up his/her position of neutrality.

Several traps threaten the success of therapy:

1. Siding with the patient who has "been made ill by his/her family." In this case, the therapist adheres to a one-dimensional concept which makes the adolescent the victim of pathogenic parents. This is an underestimation of the enormous power the adolescent has at his/her disposal in the role of a consenting victim: in this role, he/she permanently figures in the parents' emotional and educational failure in relation to him/her and increases their guilt. A therapeutic strategy of this kind accelerates the escalation of mutual aggressions between the adolescent and his/her parents.
2. This is also the case when the therapist serves as a spokesperson for the "rebellious" adolescent by decoding, in a simplistic manner, the young person's behavior problems as manifestations of resistance. The therapist thereby hides the transgenerational dimension of the symptom (a frequent fascination on the part of the parents for deviance or illness) and its latent meaning: in fact, the adolescent, beyond the immature conventions and protestations that he/she adopts, gets more and more deeply involved in a logic of dependence. The establishment of a secret alliance with the adolescent designated as patient is, above all, sometimes the case with young therapists who replay, within the framework of family interviews, the missed steps of their own separation – individuation process.
3. On the other hand, older therapists have a tendency to place themselves in either an open alliance or competition or rivalry with the adolescent's parents. Both of these attitudes, if they are repetitious, increase the risks of disqualifying the therapist when either are considered to be present by the adolescent or his/her parents.

Recourse to co-therapy or supervision appreciably reduces these risks during the course of therapy.

One of the theoretical bases on which most family therapists seem to be in agreement is Ludvig von Bertalanffy's [17] General Systems Theory. He attempted to formulate valid principles for a different system since these principles could be biological, physico-chemical, or other. It is the members of the Palo Alto School who have presented a possible connection between this theory and family systems theory in the most structured way. These writers have defined certain properties that are valid for many open systems. Here are the most important:

1. Totality: Just as the modification of an element in a system involves a change to a system in its totality, the behavior of the family member cannot be disassociated

from the behavior of other family members – that which happens to him/her changes the entire family. If, in therapy, one cannot seem to make a change in the adolescent's behavior, changing the parent's behavior will often have indirect effect, ultimately resulting in a change in the adolescent's behavior.

2. Non-somatization: Just as a system is not the sum of these elements, one cannot reduce a family down to the sum based on each one of its members. In the example of the conjugal system, to paraphrase the mathematicians, there are the systematic theories of "1 + 1 = 3," so "I + Thou = 3." Thus, if one considers the two parents and the adolescent, we come up with "6"!
3. Equifinality: The equifinality of like elements can be linked to initial elements which are different. This does not mean that the first years of life have no importance in relation to the individual's future, but experiences that have been gone through cannot be simplistically reduced to being the direct cause of a later problem: it is necessary to study in each case the a whole the human system in which the problem has arisen. Therefore, one definitively rids oneself of the automatic images of a rejecting or overly-possessive mother and a too-severe or too-frequently absent father as the cause of all one's unhappiness!
4. Homeostasis: Retroaction and homeostatic control make up a special class of self-regulated systems and adoptive phenomena. This element of homeostasis has been often used in systems psychotherapy. In 1957, Don B. Jackson [18] advanced a hypothesis according to which the patient's illness could be understood as a homeostatic mechanism having as its function the bringing back into balance of a family system in danger of changing.

We evoke the example of an adolescent whose school, anorectic, or drug addiction problems happen to be blocking their change but which also, at the same time, prevent the redefining of his/her parents' marital relationship.

Paradoxical prescriptions for change flush out then that which works because one belongs to a certain family system: "It's very important that you remain a child for the time being because I feel that you're very worried about having to help your parents who might not be ready yet to find themselves again as a couple…" These kind of comments, which certainly come out of what has been said by patients in sessions, brings about not only a certain confusion in the adolescent who believed him/herself to be in an out-and-out rebellion against his/her parents, but also a crisis with his/her parents who will inevitably find themselves to be forced to show that the two of them can go out by themselves and that they can derive pleasure from one another as a couple.

5. The Systems Model of Health Problems: The Founding Fathers

We should immediately remark that with systems theory, the founding fathers are not to be considered icons or objects to be worshiped. They propose certain theoretical models leading to practice applications that demonstrate a certain kind of effectiveness. Every new school of therapy can be draw upon them while developing its own creative ideas.

From the systems theory perspective, dysfunctional relationships between an adolescent and his/her many environments (family, professional, the community) can contribute to the genesis of psychosomatic illnesses. More frequently, one can state that a somatic attack is maintained and perpetuated by contextual factors which then contribute to the risk for chronification. Said differently, we are going to take an interest in using the family system and relational dynamics such that they can alter any symptom, starting at the moment that it is used as a means of communicating. Thus, as an example, a child's seasonal asthma attack is in the first place simply a poor adaptation to a stimulus that might be physical in nature. But if it is reinforced by the mother's anxiety, or if she allows the child to quickly see from the start that this attack functions as an antagonism of the parental couple's problems because it forces the parents to reunify, this attack runs the risk of repeating itself or becoming chronic while provoking and rigidifying an interactional cycle.

The majority of family therapists have taken up the possible reading of a somatic symptom in terms of communication problems. Therefore, Mr. Bowen [19] observes the clinical contexts in which everything happens as if the soma of one family member reflects the psyche of another. Thus, a little girl's enuretic symptoms have the effect of diverting all of her mother's attention which distracts and turns her, in a circular manner, away from her initial anxiety which was centered on another object (the grandmother's illness) prior to the enuretic episodes. In the domain of somatic medicine in relation to family therapy, the most elaborate and best known model came out of the work of Salvator Minuchin and his team in Philadelphia which is published in his book entitled "Psychosomatic Families." [20] The model was elaborated, starting with the evaluation of a family that included a child or adolescent overcome by disorders like asthma, chronic abdominal pain, diabetes, and anorexia. With hyperlabile diabetics and unstable asthmatics, Minuchin made certain specifics known: in these families, attention is essentially centered around the child which thus ensures a regulation of the interpersonal relationship between the couple. They noted the following family/characteristics as those which are considered typical of families with psychosomatic interactions:

1. They have a certain type of family organization and interaction.
2. The child is involved in parental conflicts.
3. The child is physiologically vulnerable (this point is very important because it is not a matter of it being "all psychological").

We shall go into detail on the first two points which constitute the original contribution by the Minuchin team.

The type of family organization and interactions goes back to the following elements: the entanglement of relationships and their rigidity are accompanied by an omnipresent worry about protection that each family member has in relation to the others while the same results in a chronic non-resolution of conflicts. The absence of a boundary between the generations and their roles prevents the disengagement of the individual in relation to his/her family. The lack of adaptation to both external and internal stimuli maintains the status quo when a change in customary interactions would be necessary, like at the time a child moves into adolescence. Finally, the lack of negotiating behavior, which is always reported, reinforces this mechanism even more.

These characteristics, which have to be placed along a continuum, vary in their intensity, depending on the family. They are described in more detail as follows:

- Enmeshement of relationships with an overinvestment of some members in relation to others, and interference in relaying communications (a grandmother in the role of parent, a child making adult decisions, etc.). If one family member laughs, they all start to laugh. One of them may respond in the place of another. The roles and the behaviors of each one of them are hardly differentiated.
- Overprotection: Each protects the other, but essentially on the basis of a conjugal, concrete plan, while not recognizing the emotional dimension.
- Rigidity: Family rules are not to be broken and are immutable, from one generation to the next. Capacities for adaptation to change are limited – thus, one will see the parents of older adolescents continuing to behave with them like they used to when these children were young. The elements of experience are moments of fragility: symptoms appear at the time of a death, marriage or birth, or what is more usual, at the time when the child moves out of the family home. This involves, as one example, a change of distance in relation to the families of origin.
- Non-resolution of conflicts: The most important family rule is the following: "We are a family where everyone sees everything in the same way." From this point of view, a state of internal fusion and isolation from the outside results. Therefore, dark feelings on account of any disagreement seem disloyal vis-à-vis the family. No one expresses his/her disagreement: one consciously represses it. If the darkness caused by tensions might appear, it could be displaced by one's interest being directed, for example, at the illness of a family member since the family does not allow the expression of aggressive affect!

Involvement of the child in parental conflicts. Conflict management in these families is carried out according to several models. Pathological triangulations and privileged coalitions with the child translate into a stable alliance between one of the parents and the patient. The other parent is placed in a marginal position without the same being verbalized! The strategy of diversion, for the child, consists of short-circuiting parental conflicts and mobilizing the couple. All marital tensions and tensions with the preceding generations are annuled – the psychosomatic illness becomes the family's sole problem.

Minuchin's therapeutic model is of the structural type, that is to say, it consists of re-examining family functioning while attempting to offer the same means to redefine its structures. Therefore, it reinforces parental dynamics and stimulates circularity among all family members. For example, Minuchin will ask the parents of an anorexic to assume the responsibility themselves of demanding that their daughter eat to allow her to force the emergence of her aggressivity. He recommends this structural approach as the treatment of choice for psychosomatic ailments. Afterwards, one's role as a mediator of emotion progressively moves back towards talking. The patient can allow him/herself to recognize a meaning in relation to his/her symptoms when he/she sees his/her family's attitude change before these expressions of emotions, both positive and negative. Therefore, individual psychopathological problems are not denied by the clinician, but his/her considerable experience leads him/her to affirm that this approach to the symptom within his/her echoing system often allows him/her to release the patient from invalidating, even deadly pathologies.

Numerous practitioners, one of whom is J.H. Weakland [21], remain cautious and on guard against a one-dimensional and simplistic nosographical view that would link such familial dysfunction and psychosomatic ailment too closely together. It is important to never get tired of repeating that systems models are not etiological or explanatory models of psychosomatic disorders. It is simply a matter of a correlation between one type of family functioning and the chronification of a somatic illness when compared to control groups. The poorest functioning, in terms of communication and capacity for affective response, is perhaps the result of the poor adaptative mechanisms of families in relation to the illness of one of its members. What is important from the therapeutic point of view is an understanding of how families reorganize themselves around the problem of health and head down a one-way street towards a dead end if the solutions they adopted are themselves a source of problems. Putting a framework of security back into place (through the work of restructuring) and opening up space for talking (the expression of emotions) in a climate of empathy vis-à-vis all family members are the principal therapeutic tools using this approach. These tools will allow the family to recapture the dynamics of its destiny and will bring about the emergence of their possibilities for self-healing. The goal is for all the members of the family to recover a certain feeling of control over their lives. Therefore, the parents often become aware that the close relationship they had as a couple before they had children is no longer present and that they should find another way to be as just two. For separated couples who get back in contact with one another on the occasion of their child's illness, there is sometimes a real task of true separation to be realized. They are no longer a couple but they are still the mother and father of their child.

Drawing inspiration from the structural model is a guiding thread for the therapist that he/she can apply to new family models: there is the single-parent family, the reconstituted family, the host family, and the "institutional family" (there is sometimes a lively competition between the institutional structures and biological parents…). In 1985, Stierlin [22] had already broadened the typology of families that have psychosomatic interactions by identifying 3 types of at-risk families:

1. Close-knit families: They represent the majority of families with psychosomatic transactions and correspond in large part to the families described by Minuchin: they are victims of obligatory familial harmony. They refuse to get involved in conflict and they demonstrate too much solicitude within the sphere of the concrete. The family is so close-knit that there is unresolved work of mourning and non-negotiation regarding separations.
2. Divided families: These represent a third of all psychosomatic families, and with them, only a single part of their system is united in harmony: as an example, the mother and her sick child who are in a stable coalition against the father. The child is bound to the good parent against the bad parent. A lot of adolescents find themselves confronted again by the fact that they themselves have to deal with their parents' problems and push away the parent to whom they find themselves bound in order to get way from the other parent. This will be a terrible debt to pay when they themselves will want to become part of a couple.

3. Families in dissolution: They are most often described as being in the group of families that consists of carriers of psychological or psychopathic disorders. One finds an exceptional amount of sick adolescents in this type of family.

We obviously cannot omit here the contribution on Mara Selvini [23] of Milan who carried out some remarkable observational work and who proposed therapeutic outlines for families of anorexics. She emphasizes the escalation of sacrifices and the "conspiracy of silence" in these families which prevent any expression of agressivity other than the refusal to eat. These interventions attempt to give rise to revolt and indignation on the part of the sick one, comportment that Selvini is, paradoxically, very pleased with while designating it as a behavior which allows the adolescent to remain a little girl for her parents for a long time. Selvini thus attempts to replace passive violence with the start of a verbal protest by reframing the eating problem as an adolescent crisis. Therefore, one sees that the work of family therapy consists of making the family system move towards a critical phase designated as "bifurcation" [24] beyond which a change of direction of the condition can be put into scope in relation to issues that are not a priori foreseeable. Such an interpretation, which demonstrates the positive aspects of an "adolescent crisis," will orient the therapist towards researching the progressive potentialities of the system in view of the patient's expressed suffering, whatever it might be, and will allow him/her to adopt a different attitude in the emergency room other than that of putting a stop to the crisis, at any cost, through attempting to return the adolescent to a previous state that was a pre-pathological condition (cf. Adolescents at Emergency Room, V. Dubois, in this book).

6. Family Systems Therapy Makes Use of Tools which Could Be of Use in Medicine

We have demonstrated the utility of a family systems approach for health problems with adolescents who are blocked in their stage of change. Without being a therapist, every caregiver and doctor will have an interest in utilizing the systems' tools which could be valuable to the latter, particularly in the case of non-requesting patients or those who often have disorganized and idiosyncratic kinds of contact with family members. It is also a matter of not making the patient feel guilty.

a) The "non-requesting patient"
The physician is often confronted with clinical situations in which his/her client does not initially appear to be asking for care or changes, at least on a verbal level. The subject only rarely appears to be the sole bearer of the request, which does not mean that he might not actually have a request.

Perhaps a general practitioner will ask for the patient to meet with a psychiatrist or a psychologist when the somatic adolescent patient, which is often the case, will not take this step him/herself. The systems approach proves to be extremely useful in that case since the consulting psychiatrist or psychologist can initiate dialogue with the adolescent. Through metacommunicating (communication on top of another communication) at the request of the initial physician (but for what reason, in your opinion, would the doctor on duty have requested a psychiatric opinion?), our "client" will then actually be those who actually constitute the relationship between the adolescent and the doctor. Going back to the family, we know that the adolescent, even when suffering, does not perceive such a relationship as pertinent and even finds it humiliating to look for outside help. The parents are often worried. A systems perspective will allow us then to call upon the adolescent by asking him/her to help us help his/her parents. This very advantageous position often allows one to reopen a space for dialogue. This method is extremely useful in medicine because, other than the fact that it allows for an organized and quick collection of a heteroanamnesis carried out in the presence of the patient, it allows for the resituating of the illness's course in the patient's history and in the family history. In addition, the presence of members from the family circle permit that the benefits of the intervention are not solely restricted to obtaining information.

In the example of the asthmatic adolescent cited above, it would therefore be desirable for him/her to become aware that the therapist is taking into consideration the role that he/she plays, in spite of him/herself, in his/her asthma attacks: it is a reconciliatory role in relation to his/her parents who are in conflict. If this reframing is formulated in front of the parents, the child and the family members, along with the therapist, can put an alternative strategy into place regarding the asthma attacks to reassure the child in such a way so that he/she will no longer have the need to resort to them in order to see his/her parents show their solidarity again. Thus, according to Minuchin, a structural intervention would consist of asking both parents to come in for consultation so that they can discuss their problems together without sifting through the discourse that their children have generated. Mara Selvini might add that perhaps there should be a more stringent intervention with the child by informing him/her that its not up to children to occupy themselves with settling their parents' problems, that they are not their parents' mother or father, and that they have their own life as an adolescent to carry out.

It is very obvious that such reframings with somatic patients are only possible when a sufficiently stable relationship conducive to trust has been able to be established. If the patients do not initiate any verbalizations, we prefer a cautious attitude in regard to the same while respecting the denial of emotions and the difficulties they may have in verbalizing transactions. The therapist can then close him/herself up inside of the system by making an extensive alliance with the patient. For example, one could propose that the mother do more about moving just slowly towards the point of bifurcation in relation to the care of her child by making up her mind on her own that she's had enough of attending to her older adolescent's needs and that she wants to make some time for just herself and her husband. If the father is present during the session, one can also expect that he will express how he feels excluded and the therapist will explain how he can initiate a recapturing of the most intimate kinds of contact with his wife.

b) The notion of circular causality as an inducing agent of non-guilt in the therapeutic process.

   We see way too often, above all with psychological problems, causal one-dimensional interpretations of the following type: "Our son has problems at school because my husband is never home!" A systemic view of the situation allows us to not take sides and to not look for a guilty party since causality is to be found in communicational misunderstandings. In our Western world, it is difficult to make a departure from this etiological research which is, however, not very useful from the therapeutic point of view. We should think about how somatic practitioners send their patients, in particular, adolescents, to a psychiatrist: "It's his/her nerves; it's all in his/her head." A lower-level position on the matter is really more useful: "We will try to find a solution together and I would like to have my psychiatrist colleague's opinion regarding all the problems that you have all been aware of as far as stress factors that might have a role in the illness."

7. Clinical Vignettes

Gregory, 17, has developed obesity and has had problems at school over the last year. We learn in passing that his father left his mother a year ago and that she is in a very depressed auto- and heteroaggressive mode. She wants a lot from her husband who abandoned her after 25 years of marriage and about the same from her son whom she doesn't hesitate to lash out at by saying, "You're just like your father!" A fact that is more serious than that is that the mother has made several suicide attempts. Our young patient has given up his social life, and most notably vacations with friends, because he appears to have a social phobia. During an interview where he was present with his mother, he expressed, in a highly emotional state, that he doesn't want to leave the house because he's afraid that he will find his mother dead upon his return.

When the mother becomes aware of the therapist's role and of how she had indeed involuntarily turned her son into a scapegoat, she was able to adopt a calmer attitude. Unfortunately, in this case, it is not yet possible to have both parents in a session together because their breakup still entails too much anger and bitterness. Therefore, we opted for two alternating interviews, one time with the mother and one time with the father.

Thomas, 18, is a Korean child who was adopted when he was very young by an idealistic couple who had gone through the maze of medical examinations and treatments for sterility. Thomas is the couple's second adoptive child – it was carried out a little bit so that he could be company for his brother, and a little bit so that the couple could become a true family. During the course of the ups and downs of emotional events, the adoptive mother was found to be hyperinvested in Thomas. She was the perfect mother while the father was becoming uninvested in the family unit in favor of a certain degree of alcoholism and extramarital affairs. When he was 18, Thomas made a series of repeated suicide attempts based on mystical and philosophical themes having to do with the meaning of life. The situation could not be stabilized until the moment when, during their family interviews, the therapist was able to evoke Thomas's foreign origins, his desire to see his country again, and perhaps find traces of his biological parents again. This was a test for the adoptive parents, but at the same time, the bonds between them grew stronger. In taking charge of the situation, we were able to propose individual interviews with the adolescent, concurrently with family sessions and couple's sessions for the parents in which they were able to approach their own problems, including those in the sexual sphere.

Vincent, 20, after a few attempts to separate from the family at the time of adolescence, returned back to the family cocoon. He suffers from disabling gastric ulcers. Vincent states, "There is nothing better than having a family like mine. We always agree on everything because we all feel the same. And if one of us is sad, we all become sad. I would rather go on vacation with my family than with my friends." Vincent's father never grows tired of bragging about all of his son's virtues: he courageous and wise, he studies a lot, and he doesn't do anything stupid.

The mother completes the picture by bringing up Vincent's kind and affectionate nature. Accordingly, Vincent earns his parents' approval. He occupies a central place in the family, leaving his brothers and sisters on the periphery. He is the mediator between all the members of the family. He is the reservoir for and gathers, stabilizes and prevents tensions and possible conflicts. In spite of his apparent fagility (he is sick!), Vincent rules over the entire life of the family members. Meals are served at a precise hour, the dishes are chosen based on his diet, and everyone observes silence so as not to disturb the sick one's rest.

The actual harmony of the family, at the cost occasioned by the illness, is a reflection of the harmony that reigned in Vincent's parents' families of origin. In effect, Vincent's mother has taken on the role of a caretaking wife by surrounding a progressively disabled husband, who contracted multiple sclerosis very early on, with care. Vincent's father had experienced the loss of a younger brother and his mourning had marked the family atmosphere by reinforcing attachment bonds. With this family where there is typical psychosomatic interaction, the work has progressed slowly only when the parents have been able to bring up their own ambivalence with regard to attachment, but also, slowly in regard to that sadness that reigns in their own family, so that possible new behaviors might make themselves known to Vincent. Consequently, the ulcer attacks have been less frequent.

8. Conclusion

We have seen that the family systems approach can be harmoniously integrated with the general medical and psychiatric approaches as adjuncts for complex and problematic situations that surround adolescent health problems. We believe that this contributes to a better understanding and treatment of resistant cases that present intricacies in family functioning in relation to the obtaining of benefits from this relational type.

For years, with traditional medicine having perhaps suffered from seeing the psychological and psychopathological approaches center excessively on intrapsychic processes to the detriment of what is concrete and present, we have wanted to emphasize how easily family therapy registers in the "there and then," while also taking into account somatic symptoms that are, above all, spoken about with difficulty.

The notion of circular causality brings about a non-blaming clinical approach and allows a great opening up towards solutions that are sometimes unexpected. It allows us to go beyond binary logics that too often surround adolescent problems. Ideas based on the systems approach can be applied like those used inside of strict family therapy, but any medical approach can be draw from systems theory.

Every physician, from the moment a problem becomes complex, has an interest in proceeding with focusing in on the problem and analyzing the symptom's location, not only in relation to the psychic economy of the subject, but also as regards his/her function in the larger system. This attitude in relation to the patient is very respectful because the practitioner automatically transmits to him/her information learned from other family members. It also lets one inform and support the other members of the family. We will no longer look at the family in a blaming way, but with interest. They are a source of information for us and a social support for the patient. Furthermore, in the clinical setting we will often see that the parents of our suffering adolescents are suffering even more than their child and really need comprehensive attention from medical personnel.

It seems to us that, without actually wanting to do so, we have demonstrated that family systems therapy should be a part of every caregiver's coursework and should be fully integrated into medical studies! All doctors are, in effect, confronted by maladaptive reactions to stress from illness in dysfunctional families. Therefore, they should, at the least, be rather sensitive to these chronification factors in order to know how to make a departure from one-dimensional causal reasoning and they should collaborate with a family therapist, psychologist, or psychiatrist. Many interventionists will be anxious to reform a family system with clear and complementary relationships which resonate! A psychologist can certainly propose a psychotherapeutic treatment that is an adjunct to standard medical treatment for he/she is concerned not only with the corpus of the family, but also with the patient's biological body which is suffering.

This same systems approach would likewise be very useful to us for analyzing the relationships between generalist and specialist physicians, and the diverse interventionists surrounding the patient. Such an approach would bring us professional social support that would be susceptible to protecting us from "burn-out," [25].

Reflecting on these issues is not a luxury that to be added onto the practice of medicine. It is really a caregiving approach to increase therapeutic effectiveness.

Between the "flight into the future" with technology, which is always more and more difficult to understand, and the attraction of healers, gurus, and magician of every sort, there is always a place for a responsible physician who is concerned with the link between biological dysfunction and family dysfunction in relational transactions, and between bodily suffering and family suffering.

References

[1] Selvini-Palazzoli. Self Starvatuin. Aronson, New-York, 1974.

[2] Whitaker C.A., Blumberry W.M. Dancing with the family. *A symbolic experiential approach,* Brunner/Mazel, 1988.

[3] Richardson H.B. Patients have families, N.Y. *Commonwealth Fund,* 1948.

[4] Reynaert Ch., Janne P., Mortreu B., Melange M., Debongnies J.C., Mainguet P. Approche psychosomatique de l'ulcère gastro-duodénal: de la perte de contrôle chez le patient ulcéreux au contrôle médical de l'ulcère. *Louvain Méd.* 1991 ; 110: 197-202.

[5] Birraux A. Le processus d'adolescence. *Science et vie*. 1994 ; 188 : 34-46.

[6] Zdanowicz N. Un abord thérapeutique de l'adolescent par le corps ? *Psychologie Médicale*. 1994 ; 26, 13 : 1345-1347.

[7] Reynaert Ch., Verreckt E., Tordeurs D., Zdanowicz N., Van Houtte M.. La vie affective et sexuelle après 50 ans. Belgian Journal for Sexual Health, décembre 2004 ; 1 : 12-17.

[8] d'Alcantara A., Van Meerbeeck Ph. Peau d'âmes : *quelles médiations pour l'adolescence ?* In De Boeck-Université, Bruxelles, 1991.

[9] Godenir F., Algrain V., Verrekt E., Zdanowicz N., Reynaert Ch. Adolescents en danger, parents en difficulté...*Louvain Médical,* septembre 2005 ; 124 (7) : 286-292.
[10] Zdanowicz N., Janne P., Reynaert Ch. Family, health and adolescence. *Psychosomatic.* 2004 ; 45 : 500-507.
[11] Zdanowicz N., Reynaert Ch. Adolescent health. *The Lancet.* 2004 ; 364 : 247.
[12] Reynaert Ch. « Météo couple ». *Année de la Famille. Louvain.* 2004 ; 45 : 15-19.
[13] Stierlin H. Separating parents and adolescents. Jason Aronson, New-York 1981.
[14] Bateson G., Jackson D. Some varieties of pathogenic organization. In David McK. Rioch et Weinstein, eds., Disorders of communication, Research Publications. Association for research in nervous and mental diseases, Baltimore, William and Wilkins 1964 ; Vol 42 : p.270-83 ; trad. Fr. dans Bateson, vers une écologie de l'esprit, T. II., Paris Seuil, 1972.
[15] Watzlawick P. Une logique de la communication. Paris, Seuil, 1972.
[16] Stierlin H. Countertransference in family therapy with adolescents in the adolescent in group and family therapy. *Max Sugar.* Brunner-Malzel. New-York, 1975.
[17] von Bertalanffy L. General system theory, New-York. Georges Braziller, 1968. Trad. Franç. J.B. Chabrol : *Théorie générale des systèmes.* Dunod, Paris, 1973.
[18] Jackson D.D. The question of family homeostasis. *Psychiatric Quarterly Supplement,* 1ère partie, 1957 ; 31 : 79-90.
[19] Bowen M. The use of family theory in clinical practice. *Compr. Psychiat.* 1966 ; 7 : 3-45.
[20] Minuchin S., Rosman B.L., Baker L. Psychosomatic families : anorexia nervosa in context, Cambridge Mass. Harvard University Press, 1978.
[21] Weakland J.H. 1974. « Somatique familiale » : une marge négligée. Trad. de l'américain, in *« Sur l'interaction ».* Le seuil, Paris, 1981, pp.456-472.
[22] Wirsching M., Stierlin H. Psychosomatics I. Psychosocial characteristics of psychosomatic patients and their families ». *Family systems medicine.* 1985 ; 3 : 6-17.
[23] Selvini-palazzoli M. Self-starvation : from the intrapsychic to the transpersonal approach of anorexia nervosa. *Human Context Books.* London, 1974.
[24] Elkaim M. Si tu n'aimes ne m'aime pas. *Approche systémique et psychothérapie.* Seuil 1989, p.45.
[25] Reynaert Ch., Libert Y, Janne P., Zdanowicz N. Comment allez-vous, Docteur ? Le burn-out du médecin. *Louvain Méd.* 2001 ; 120 n° 9: 296-310.

In: The Adolescent Today in Medicine
Editors: N. Zdanowicz, et al. pp. 89-124
ISBN: 978-1-60021-764-7

Chapter 7

THE ADOLESCENT IN FAMILY MEDICAL PRACTICE

P. Eeckeleers[*]
General Medicine, Scientific Association of General Medicine

ABSTRACT

It is important to keep in mind that the adolescent expects a non-paternalistic, non-judgmental, respectful relationship with his/her treating physician. He/She asks for information, but paradoxically, the messages of prevention are hardly ever integrated by him/her.

The family physician should systematically broaden the scope of the initial consultation, not only to look into specific medical problems (acne, dysmenorrhea, amenorrhea, growth disorders, dorsolumbar pain, appearance of chronic illnesses, etc.) and masked sufferings (academic failure, behavior disorders, drug additions, in general, etc.), but also to deliver messages for important prevention (STD's, alcohol, tobacco, sports or other types of accidents). The adolescent hardly ever consults with his/her family doctor. When he/she does consult with the doctor, it is mainly for common infectious or trauma disorders. Booster vaccinations and requests for sports fitness certificates are likewise other reasons for consultation.

An adolescent who is not well only rarely goes to the doctor on his/her own initiative: he/she is often brought to a consultation by his/her worried parents. This consultation does not unfold easily, whether the adolescent is soothed by the fact that his parents are worried and brings him/her to us or whether (which is markedly more frequent) he/she clams up, associating us with the hostile world of adults. But the doctor will have to conduct the interview in order to, from the start, objectify the suffering while looking for the alarm signals of depression or suicidal ideation, preferably when the adolescent does not have his/her parents present. It will be indispensable to differentiate between an actual problem of depression, that may or may not entail at-risk behaviors or a risk of suicide, and the simple incidence of depression that is associated with the experience of adolescence itself.

[*] Contact: P. Eeckeleers, rue de Rochefort 40, 5590 Leignon (Belgium) Tél : 003283215492 Fax : 003283215492, E.mail : ricardo.muniz@win.be

Keywords: GP, adolescents, prevention.

1. Introduction

The child that the family doctor often follows from his/her most tender infancy has grown. At the time of the last consultation, the adolescent was still a child and he/she now presents him/herself before the doctor as a young man or a young woman, often a bit ill-at-ease. At the time of the clinical examination, the practitioner lowers him/herself down to the level of the adolescent to examine him/her. It is now the doctor who must lower him/herself…

But if the difference is noticeable to the adults who have watched the child grow, it is necessary to realize that he/she is not the same as he/she was; his/her expectations regarding the doctor are different. He/she demands that the doctor respect him/her and what he/she says, while still always needing support from an adult, whether it be his/her parent, a teacher, and even his/her doctor.

1.1. Why Speak Specifically about the Role of the Family Doctor?

As will be explained further on, adolescents rarely consult with a doctor. It just so happens that these rare consultations are, at the least, opportunities for the doctor to reestablish contact and to make a quick assessment which is not only medical and preventative, but also for the purpose of screening adolescents who are suffering and possibly at risk for suicide. The general practitioner is often the first paramedical interventionist called out to, whether it be by the adolescent him/herself or by a referring adult. This is, without a doubt, tied in with the doctor's psycho-medical-social knowledge of adolescence, but also because of his/her extensive availability.

From a recent paper presented at the WONCA[1] Congress in Florence during August of 2006 [2], it was pointed out once again that general practitioners are, on account of their holistic and centered approach to the patient, in a particularly good position to screen, take charge of, and treat problems that crop up in the adolescent population. Adolescent malaise does not necessarily require that a doctor take charge of the situation. On the contrary, this might have a deleterious effect. Indeed, many problems tied into adolescence are not meant to be medicalized: listening; empathy, dialogue and the neutral offering of information are, in many cases, enough to play down their importance and get them resolved. Moreover, as a study recently carried out in Belgium demonstrates, adolescents themselves consider the family doctor their primary resource person in the event of a medical or other problem.

[1] WONCA: World Organization of National Colleges, Academies and Academic Associations of General Practioners/Family Physicians.

1.2. Interest in Action Targeted at the Adolescent Group

In the domain of public health, priorities for action mainly have to do with obesity prevention, tobacco addiction, sexually transmitted diseases (STD's), and pregnancy prevention. These priorities have been the same for the last 20 years. On the other hand, the prevalence of chronic diseases has increased in the adolescent population whether it be, for example, asthma or diabetes.

The adolescent mortality rate has generally diminished less rapidly than the pediatric mortality rate, as a result of the increase in fatal injuries and suicides in the former group. In the United Kingdom, the mortality rate from injuries and suicides has increased from the 11% total mortality rate of adolescents between the years 1901 and 1910 to 57% in 2003 [4].

At-risk behaviors (alcohol consumption, drugs, delinquency) contribute to the creation of social and medical disparities during the transition from adolescence to adulthood. Unfortunately, these differences persist throughout adulthood. In effect, there clearly exists a stronger correlation between an adolescent's health and his/her health in adulthood than between his/her health of childhood and that of his/her adolescence.

In 2002, an English study [5] showed that 11-15 year-old youths who smoke regularly had three times as many alcohol-related problems and six times the number of serious psychological problems in adulthood than those who did not.

Therefore, adolescence is a critical period from which the number of learned behaviors will persist into adulthood and have a lasting influence on one's health. At first glance, effective medical interventions will have to recognize the existence of multiple health problems that are specific to adolescence.

2. Conducting Consultations with Adolescents in General Practice

The initial consultation should begin by centering on the problem set forth by the young person so that he/she is convinced of the physician's recognition of and interest in his/her problem. This can afterwards be extended to other areas.

Whatever the reason announced for the consultation at the beginning by the adolescent, it could be the pretext for a first meeting that will allow him/her to reveal the actual problem that brings him/her there. That might be the only patient/doctor contact if he/she feels he hasn't been listened to. Therefore, it is a matter of the doctor being attentive.

As for any patient, the doctor will take care to practice effective medicine while endeavoring to evaluate his/her physical, psychological, and social health (food, housing, environment, vocational), according to the WHO's definition of the same. The young person should be able to perceive that his/her family doctor can be a good resource if he/she finds him/herself in a difficult situation.

A high quality adolescent/doctor relationship, is of great importance for it will allow for an alliance regarding therapeutic options to develop and will also be favorable for the patient's taking into account of the preventative messages delivered by the physician.

Throughout the consultation, the practitioner will take care to make the young person feel secure while at the same time making him/her aware of his/her responsibilities.

2.1. Management of Third Parties

Relatively speaking, the adolescent often has someone with him during his consultation, most of the time his/her mother.

The presence of a third party can be a burden for this young person for if the former imposes him/herself on the situation, he/she will not allow the adolescent to express him/herself freely. But his/her presence can also be reassuring. Some young women still come to their consultations accompanied by their mothers, up until the time they are about twenty years old. And likewise many young people come the first time accompanied by a friend. Therefore, it is important to know what is the place and role of this third party in the patient's life, but also, who is the one actually asking for contact with the physician.

One musn't overlook the fact either that some parents are extremely anxious vis-à-vis their child and that this is also a matter of reassuring them. On the other hand, the systematic absence of a third party, above all in the case of the youngest children, can be a sign of parental neglect.

If the consultation might eventually be carried out with the presence of a third party, the doctor should not hesitate, if he/she deems it necessary, to have the third party leave during the course of the consultation. The consultations that follow should be carried out without the latter.

2.2. Approaching the Adolescent

It is important to put the family physician's intervention into its true perspective. Even if many adolescents resent their need to be "mothered," the doctor should resist the temptation to play the part of parent with these patients. Along the same line of thought, as much as the adolescent is looking for a friendly or meaningful relationship with the doctor, he cannot consider him/her as a friend or companion who is giving advice. The family doctor should present him/herself as a competent and responsible professional, an empathetic adult with whom the adolescent patient can talk, and a support who is capable of turning him/herself into the adolescent's spokesperson by defending his/her genuine preoccupations [7]. It is extremely important that, from the moment the young person enters the doctor's office, he/she feels respected as a responsible person.

And this should be the case even if the physician consulted is usually the one chosen by his/her parents, someone whom the young person has sometimes known since earliest childhood.

2.2.1. What Are the Main Elements that Make the Adolescent Ill-at-Ease with the Doctor?

Adolescents are sometimes embarrassed when they run into people whom they know in the waiting room, particularly if they come on their own initiative.

- Waiting their turn is unbearable for some of them.
- The cost of the consultation can put a stop to things if their parents or guardian don't know about it or if they do not assume the financial responsibility for it.

- A lot of adolescents think that doctors have the right to divulge the content of the consultation to their legal guardian.
- A certain proportion of adolescents do not feel confident when they are in front of their family doctor (a). Specifically, 1 out of 3 girls, and 13% of boys feel very ill-at-ease [3]. This feeling is exacerbated when the doctor is male and increases even more at the time of the clinical examination.
- The medical jargon seems incomprehensible to the adolescents and causes them to be afraid. This language gives them the impression that they have not been listened to or understood. The practitioner should keep this basic knowledge in mind, which means that the following questions should sometimes be asked at the start:
- Do your parents know about your coming here?
- Do you want to arrange a consultation with one another rather than a regular appointment?
- Is the cost of the visits a problem?
- If the answer is "yes," that should not be an obstacle: a solution should be found.

In addition, the issue of medical confidentiality should be clarified: medical confidentiality is implicitly understood and absolute in the case of children.

It is important to be constantly reformulating the adolescent's words through the use of common language so that he/she feels heard and understood.

2.2.2. Criteria for Choosing a Physician

The personality and motivation of the physician are clearly more important than his/her training.

From the initial moments of the consultation, the adolescent will be able to perceive if his doctor is ill-at-ease or uptight in his role, or if conversely, the latter brings all the requested attention into the consultation with the necessary overtures required by the him/her. If the relationship is good, adolescents will like meeting with their physician to talk to him/her about their problems. On the other hand, in the at-risk group of young people, 60% judged the doctor as being too quiet and not very curious in their relationship with them. 45% (30% of young people in general) did not express all that they wanted to during the consultation because of not feeling confident enough to do so. In addition, 23% of these at-risk youths had the impression that their questions were not really answered.

2.2.3. The Physician's Attitude

In French, as well as in other languages, the use of the formal "you" is a sign of respect and distance as opposed to the use of the more familiar form of "you." Although it may be difficult for the physician to use the formal form of "you" in front of the adolescent whom he has followed since earliest childhood, it is necessary, in spite of everything, to go along with this course of action. This is clearly more obviously so as far as a new, young patient is concerned. It is important to demonstrate to the young patient that we respect him/her and consider him/her to be a autonomous and responsible person.

2.2.3.1. "The Three C's"

As stated before, it is imperative that one respects "The Three C's:" confidentiality, informed consent, and counseling.

Confidentiality: Reassure the adolescent regarding the confidentiality of all that is said during the consultation. It is essential to establish a method of communication for contact and therapeutic results (via text messaging?)

Informed Consent: The adolescent often considers the taking of the medical history and, above all, the clinical examination, aggressive actions. One must bear this in mind when asking him/her for his/her authorization and when explaining the reasons for our questions and examinations to him/her.

Counseling: A good time to deliver message of prevention is during a routine examination or sports fitness examination so that the adolescent may obtain whatever certificate (for sports, vocational training, etc.) he/she needs, or at the time of a scheduled vaccination. In effect, there is no other health concern at that time and he/she will be more receptive to messages of prevention.

It is imperative to say at least once to the adolescent, and possibly even eventually in front of one of his/her parents, that we are bound to maintaining medical confidentiality, even as far as the parents, the school, or any other authority are concerned. In effect, 10% of adolescents are ignorant of this fact and they think that because they are minors, the doctor has the right, if not the duty, to repeat to the authority in charge the content of what he/she has said. It so happens that this is a basic notion in their eyes [10-11]. This confidentiality cannot obviously be always realized because 2 out of 3 consultations are not with the adolescent alone [3]: although the mother (at 44% of the consultations) or the father (at 10%) are the ones that accompany him/her to the appointments the most, siblings or acquaintances are also often present (8%).

Respect also comes about through objective and benevolent listening to what the adolescent has a sense of having respect for his/her opinions. A non-judgmental attitude, without paternalism, moralizing, or using threats or lies is imperative.

The doctor should take care to reassure the child about what he/she still is and give him/her a sense of responsibility in relation to the adult he/she is developing into.

His/her discourse should not be interrupted but it can be helped along with questions that are more or less directed towards a goal. This line of action is often useful for reformulating what the patient has just said and to assure oneself that they have comprehended well, but also for making him/her aware of things. This should be done in clear and comprehensible language. The doctor's patience is important. Some young people need time to accept surrendering themselves to treatment. This is why the physician shouldn't hesitate to agree to a quick follow-up meeting to give the adolescent time to talk, while knowing that there is also a risk that he/she will not return.

2.3. Reasons for Consultations

Few studies have been published regarding adolescents' reasons for consulting with a doctor. A study recently carried out in the waiting rooms of general practitioners offices in France and Belgium was published in 2004 [3]. The following data are mainly extracted from this study.

From the adolescent point of view, the family doctor is the primary professional resource for dialogue when there is a health problem. 85% of adolescents consulting with a general practitioner are a part of the latter's established group of patients. When someone accompanies the adolescent, it is most often the mother (44% of the time), and more rarely so the father (10%).

Girls seek out a consultation more often than boys do (57% versus 43%), mainly in the older age group bracket. The higher frequency levels of consultation are also found in the adult female population [12].

2.3.1. Why Do Young People Only Rarely Spontaneously Confide in Their Physician During Their Consultation?

A study was carried out with 9 British general practitioners: 1085 patients 18 years or older filled out a questionnaire so they could be screened for psychological disorders. Of the 258 that showed a score of disturbance, 84 were interviewed. 64 had made no mention of their problems to the doctor.

What reasons were cited for this?

- Embarrassment because of talking about the problem
- Wanting to feel they had the power to come out of the situation on their own (36%)
- Fear of annoying their physician (45%)
- A reticence tied in with the general practitioner's past or present behavior (19%). Those patients satisfaction index was not as high after the consultation

Other results given:

- Problem with the amount of time that the treatment would have taken (48%)
- The feeling that the physician would not be able to do anything about the situation (39%)
- And the feeling that the problem was not covered by the doctor (11%)

2.3.2. The Reasons Stated by Young Patients for Medical Consultations

The reasons stated ahead of time for the consultation are varied, but with identical frequency for boys as well as for girls.

Administrative and preventative reasons (certificates, vaccines), as well as respiratory problems, are most often cited (26% respectively) for both sexes.

After that come complaints having to do with their general state of health (fatigue, fever) (19%), complaints regarding their locomotor apparati (15%), digestive complaints (11%), neurological complaints (mainly headaches) (9.5%), and dermatogical complaints (acne) (5.7%).

1 out of 20 girls consult a physician for contraception issues or possible pregnancy. On the other hand, the most pressing reasons are rarely of the psychosocial type (3.8%). Older adolescents most often cite complaints of a general or respiratory nature, or issues related to contraception. Digestive complaints occur more frequently with the youngest adolescents.

To sum up, sore throats are the most frequent reason for seeking out a consultation: this involves 1 out of every 5 adolescents. The request for a doctor's certificate and illness, in the broadest sense, are the reasons for 1 out of 10 adolescents. Then come headaches and stomachaches, respectively, for less than 1 out of 10 adolescents. Vaccinations and certificates for sports are also often reasons for consultation: one out of 20 adolescents, respectively, states those reasons.

In the United States, an initial study [13] had shown that sore throats, headaches, and respiratory problems were the most frequent reasons for consultations 24% of the subjects were sexually active and 38% thought they had a weight problem. However, only 4% and 10% respectively had consulted their treating physician for these problems.

Another American study [14] found respiratory (19.4%), dermatological (10%), and osteoarticular (9.7%) complaints to be the main reasons for consultation.

A study [15] carried out by the World Health Organization (WHO) in numerous countries revealed that 30 to 40% of female adolescents complain of headaches at least once a week (versus 25% of boys of the same age). This is corroborated in part by a study [16] carried out in a Belgian school setting where weight problems and mood disorders (depression, anxiety) preoccupy 30 to 40% of adolescents. But these preoccupations are rarely put forth as the reason for consultation with their family physician.

In France, a study [17] (very limited) carried out with young people of North African descent revealed, in contrast, that the reasons for consultation were mainly on the psychosocial order (addiction, violence).

The highest frequency of consultations with older adolescent girls corresponds with requests for contraception, gyneco-obstetrical follow-ups, and preventative measures related to their sex lives.

2.3.3. Agreement with the Reasons for Consultation as Noted by the General Practitioner

According to the Belgian study mentioned previously, 80% of the reasons stated by young people have been noted and taken into account by the practitioner.

The high number of reasons that are not noted (1 out of 5) by the general physician can be interpreted in different ways:

- It could obviously have to do with a medical transcription oversight but also with not taking into account the importance of the reason for consultation in question. It is astonishing that if the adolescent often states his/her request for a certificate as the reason for the consultation, this same reason is not generally accepted by the physician as the true reason for the same. For example, a backache complaint and a request for a morning after pill might be initially limited by the patient to the backache problem when talking with the physician. Not that the contraception issue wasn't resolved, but rather that it hadn't been as important an issue with the physician.
- It can likewise be an oversight on the part of the adolescent, either a voluntary or involuntary oversight.
- The reason stated in advance by the young patient could have been a pretext because the true reason is too confidential to be written down. For example, the fear that she is pregnant or that she or he is suffering with an STD.

- The presence of a third party could have prevented the expression of a reason stated previously. For example, the need on the part of the adolescent to talk might have been noted as "rhinopharyngitis" by the physician because his/her mother was there with him/her.

But conversely, a fifth of the complaints written down by the physician hadn't been announced by the young person in the first place, such as sleep disorders, dysmenorrhea, and depression as well as other pathologies related to STD's. Likewise, unwanted pregnancies, drug dependencies, and problem drinking are rarely brought up by the young person.

Why? It is necessary to know that 1 out of 3 girls and 1 out of 7 boys does not feel comfortable with their doctor and does not dare approach certain subjects with him/her. Because of this uneasiness, this is all the more significant when the doctor is a male and at the time of a physical examination.

On the whole, hidden motives for seeking out a consultation are rare. But this is something that does show up, in spite of all the confidence a young person has in his/her physician, in general.

The doctor's professional abilities, his/her capacity for listening, the certainty of confidentiality, and his/her friendly and empathetic approach are all decisive factors for the young person who wishes to confide his/her personal problems.

2.4. Open-Ended Anamnesis

Anamnesis should, from the start, be centered on the problem brought up by the adolescent while guarding against the possibility of the problem growing wider.

A smiling and relaxed listener often allows him/herself to become interested in the patient's life and to also explore the latter's social environment, as well as his/her experiences. This will subsequently allow the doctor to broaden the scope of the consultation. The art of this lies in becoming interested in the patient's experience, while avoiding intrusiveness.

For any problem the adolescent brings up, he/she should be questioned based on his/her reaction to questions that he/she asks him/herself during the consultation, but also based on the attitudes or responses of his/her parents or friends.

To improve the screening of adolescents who are suffering, different systems of reference have been conceived (TSTS and CAFARDS) which will be detailed in the following chapter.

Anamnesis will linger on because of the frequency of adolescent problems about which, in some cases, the young person will rarely talk such as:

- Real or imaginary weight problems with the danger of irregular diets being able to lead fragile personality types into anorexic-bulimic behaviors. But there is also the problem of the commonality of televisions and computer screens in bedrooms that causes not only a lack of sleep and a lack of studying, but also weight gain, the latter being exponentially related to the number of hours spent in front of a screen.
- Nutrition problems that cause fatigue, weight gain, and insomnia: soda, greasy foods, sweets, alcohol, tobacco, etc.

- Chronic stomach pain: dysmenorrhea which is often neglected and which, however is very agonizing and disabling with certain adolescents, constipation from irregular eating habits, or somatization of a feeling of malaise.
- Headaches related to lifestyle (lack of frequent sleep, abusive consumption, etc.) or true migraines that need to be followed because they are a source of anxiety and school absenteeism, or because they originate from stress.
- Vision problems that sometimes go unrecognized.
- Pain in the cervical region of the spine, back pain, and lumbago that is sometimes of orthopedic origin, but more often related to ergonomic problems (a desk that is too low, a PC screen that is too low, an overly heavy schoolbag that is carried off to one side, etc.) or to psychosomatic problems (e.g., "having a load on one's back").
- Problems related to the genital sphere: pregnancy prevention, STD's.

2.5. The Clinical Examination: Making the Patient Feel Reassured

Adolescents need to be constantly reassured of their physical "normality." They are often very uncomfortable about their bodies which explains their embarrassment when they're undergoing a physical exam.

The doctor will take care to evaluate the patient's anxiety and take charge of the situation.

The clinical examination, often experienced as harrowing, will be commented on and explained by the physician. It will always be carried out in a gentle manner while respecting, as much as possible, any modesty on the part of the adolescent which can sometimes seem excessive.

It is important to take the following distinctive adolescent characteristics into account for whom, even if they are normal, are big sources of anxiety:

- Pubertal delays and spurts of growth, the importance of which needs to be played down.
- Gynecomastia which occurs in 1 out of 3 boys and generally disappears within 2 years.
- Mammarian asymmetry which occurs in girls (25%) and which has no pathological significance.
- Phimosis as a source of infection, which causes fear and pain at the time of sexual relations. The adolescent only rarely speaks about it. There is a risk of paraphimosis which would require an emergency procedure. Therefore, it needs to be followed.
- Real or imagined deformities, a significant source of unhappy feelings, which should be taken charge of: significant pilosity, a large nose, protruding ears, short height, breasts that are too small or too big.

3. Prevention for Adolescents

3.1. Recommended Preventative Medical Interventions

Several organizations have put forward recommendations concerning preventative examinations for adolescents who are in good health.

For adolescents, systematic screening is rarely useful. It should instead be targeted according to the young patient's lifestyle and medical history. The clinical examination, which should always be commented on and explained, allows one to reassure the adolescent about his "normality." This is an opportunity to start up a discussion about a healthy lifestyle and all its advantages.

The patient's immunization should absolutely be documented so that they can be carried out completely.

- The diphtheria-tetanus booster vaccination (adult vaccine with the smallest antidiptherial dosage) is often neglected around the age of 16. Presently, the addition of a pertussis vaccination dose is being discussed. The addition of a anti-polio booster (injectable) depends on life conditions and travel schedule, and should not be systematic.
- The status of their rubella vaccination should be verified with adolescent girls.
- The Hepatitis B vaccine, presently integrated into vaccination schedules for newborns, at least in Belgium, should ideally be administered, in the event it hasn't been already, before 15 years of age. In effect, one often forgets that in our region, Hepatitis B is not only transmitted through the blood but is a much more frequently occurring STD than AIDS, the consequences of which can be dramatic. In Belgium, since the introduction of free and systematic vaccinations for newborns, and for non-vaccinated 12-year-old adolescents, the incidence and prevalence of Hepatitis B has declined.
- The Meningoccocus C Vaccine is recommended in view of the peak of the frequency of this ailment in adolescents.
- An HPV vaccine has arrived on the market that should likewise be administered at the beginning of adolescence. In effect, the HPV virus causes cancer of the uterine cervix.

Conversation regarding the adolescent's lifestyle in general will lead to a prodigious amount of advice from the physician. The purpose of the consultation is the adolescent's well-being, both on the physical and psychological levels. This will come to pass through physical adaptation and having the feeling that he/she has control over his/her life.

So that the doctor's messages are well-perceived, it is imperative to respect certain conditions:

1. The message can never be moralizing. A simple and objective explanation will suffice. The physician must not impose requirements for behavior.
2. What the physician considers to be an at-risk behavior isn't necessarily so as far as the young person is concerned. Therefore, one must evaluate the patient's perception

of it. Moreover, that which the doctor considers a problem is sometimes considered to be a solution by the young person (smoking to slim down, drinking to amuse oneself, etc.)

3. The physician needs to make use of the young person's discomfort that is tied in with a certain behavior as a starting point to lead him/her to change the behavior.
4. It will then be a matter of accompanying the patient along with trajectory of change and helping him/her choose realistic goals.

Table 1. Preventative Intervention Recommended for Adolescents in Good Health

SCREENINGS		
	Biometric, BMI	
	Screening for static disorders (scoliosis)	
	Blood pressure	
	Screening for cervical cancer	None from the first to the 20th year, every 3 years after onset of adolescence.
	Screening for Chlamydia	If there are multiple partners.
IMMUNIZATIONS		
	Record of vaccinations	Diptheria-tetanus (dt) +/- whooping cough Polio? Chicken Pox? Hepatitis B Measles, mumps, rubella
COUNSELING		
	Nutrition and physical activity	Limitations on lipidic intake Increase of fruits and vegetable consumption Balanced caloric consumption Adequate calcium intake Regular physical activity
	Consumption	Tobacco
		Non-initiation Weaning off tobacco
	Alcohol	Limit and avoid consumption (objective information)
	Opioide substances	Recall of consumption prohibitions at time of potential at-risk behavior (driving a car, swimming, etc.)
	Sexuality (the rules of the 2 C's: conditions and contraception)	Pregnancy Prevention Prevention of STD's (protection) Avoid at-risk sexual behaviors

Adapted from: Age-specific charts, ages 11-24 years, issued by the US Preventive Services Task Force (1996 and updates), while taking into consideration some Canadian recommendations (table extracted from "L'examen médical préventif chez les adolescents: Intervenir selon leur profil de risque-Prevention en pratique médicale (TN: The Preventative Medical Examination For Adolescents: Intervention Based on At-Risk Profile-Prevention in Medical Practice), Québec, February 2005.

Problems with sleep rhythms, nutrition quality, and abusive consumption will be approached. It will be a matter of giving out clear, but non-moralistic information, by showing the possible link between certain limitations and pernicious behaviors. For example, the association between:

- tobacco abuse and limitations in running
- energy drinks and heart palpitations
- food which is too rich in sugar and fat and unexplainable feelings of being drained of energy
- stimulants and insomnia, television and significant PC use
- lack of sleep and fatigue

In these cases it is a matter is of giving the young person a sense of responsibility vis-à-vis their life choices and behaviors.

3.1.1. The Sports Fitness Examination

Frequent consultations with the family doctor are relatively rare. Therefore, every consultation should be taken advantage of to verify the adolescent's state of health. This will also take place one or two times between the ages of 12 and 18 within the framework of school medicine. The school physician likewise has a definite role in talking prevention.

One of the most frequent reasons for consultation with the family doctor consists of a request for a sports fitness certificate.

This kind of consultation should never be overlooked because, even if it seems trivial, it often allows a priori contact which is preferred for an adolescent who is in good health. It is sometimes the only yearly contact possible. It allows the physician to not only follow the young person's adequate growth, but also to evaluate his/her overall physical and mental well-being. The quality of the doctor-adolescent relationship at this time will condition the doctor's medical recourse in the event of a simultaneous or subsequent problem.

This kind of consultation is the moment of preference for carrying out prevention.

The goals of this consultation are:

- to screen for possible counter-indications for sports participation that might be foreseen and to be able to redirect the adolescent to a more appropriate sport;
- to screen and treat a pre-existing pathology, or a recent appearance of the same, that could have an influence on or could be influenced by the sport the adolescent is contemplating;
- to watch over the young sports player's growth.

3.1.2. The Anamnesis

Personal and family medical histories will be carried out because this allows the practitioner to focus his/her attention on specific risks:

- Family Medical History: sudden death, asthma, diabetes, scoliosis, heart rhythm disorders, arthritis, auto-immune disorders, significant arthrosis.
- Personal Medical History:

- Allergies, asthma
- Traumas, accidents
- Surgeries
- Orthopedic (pathologies of growth to be watched)

Treatments which are underway (or have been taken since the previous one) are sometimes unknown to the general practitioner because they are prescribed by a specialist. They shall be noted and reevaluated.

Complaints, spontaneous or non-spontaneous, that will be investigated are:

- Orthopedic pain: scoliosis, growth irregularities;
- Fatigue, weakness
- of organic origin: sideropenia in young girls, (?) post-infectious (mononucleosis, toxoplasmosis, etc.)
- those of environmental origin: sleep deficiency, excessive school work, a TV or PC in the bedroom, etc.
- those of psychosomatic origin or from a feeling of discontent: insomnia, depression, disturbing worries, etc.

The sports training involved will be quantified. It is important to quantify the significance of the physical training, keeping in mind that the sport should remain pleasurable and should therefore not bring about any a priori lesion on a growing organism that is more fragile. Young people, and boys in particular, are incapable of quantifying their effort and of listening to their bodies so that they will know their limits. Likewise, some trainers have no knowledge of the particularities of physical training in relation to growing organisms. In particular, the time that should be given over to warm-ups and stretching is not always respected because it is considered a waste of time. It just so happens that it is one of the main means for the prevention of injuries that could turn out to be serious.

On principle, one has to favor aerobic exercise (an effort of low yet prolonged intensity). On the other hand, aerobic exercise (forceful, intense, quick effort) can be increased once adolescence is over with.

3.1.3. The Clinical Examination

It is important, as stated above, to explain every medical procedure.

- Biometrics: growth is on average 6 cm per year, right up until puberty, and 10 cm per year thereafter.
- Boy's growth starts later and stretches out over a longer period.
- Pulmonary auscultation (screening for asthma through peak flow evaluation).
- Cardiac auscultation: is a murmur present?
- Otoscopy, ENT and hearing evaluations, important above all else for swimming or diving types of sports.
- Examination of vision: adjustments and evaluation for the wearing of glasses or contact lenses.
- Complete orthopedic examination:

- Search for scoliosis
- Hand-to-ground distance measurement
- Search for genu varum, genu valgum, hollow arches and flat-footedness
- Screening tests for maladies related to growth:
- Osgood Schlatter (knees)
- Scheuermann (often of the dorsal spine)
- Sever (heel)
- Oral-dental examination while insisting on the importance of hygiene at this level.
-
-

3.2. How Should the Physician Approach Prevention During the Consultation?

Few studies have been published, nor have there been many standpoints validated, regarding preventive clinical practice with adolescents, unlike for childhood or adult prevention.

A good way to undertake a quick tour of the adolescent's world is to ask him/her how it's going at home, school, with friends, and with his/her girlfriend/boyfriend.

If questions are asked in an empathetic manner about the adolescent's sports activities, pastimes (consumption of toxic substances?), his/her possible tobacco addiction, his/her sexual life (by asking about their use of contraception and preventive measures against STD's) and morals, this could likewise bring about quick responses.

3.2.1. HEADSS Questionnaire (23)

The HEADSS Questionnaire is used so that nothing will be overlooked:

- H Home
- E Education
- A Activities
- D Drugs
- S Sexuality
- S Suicide

An explicit, vague, or evasive response, as well as non-verbal responses, will allow the physician to target the problem areas following the consultation.

HEADSS: A PSYCHOSOCIAL QUESTIONNAIRE

SUGGESTION FOR STARTING THE QUESTIONNAIRE
"I would like to ask you some questions, at least if you would allow me to. You are under no obligation to answer them. But for me, this is important because it might allow me to help you. It's obvious, like I already said, that these questions will be strictly between us. The only exception would be if you or somebody else would run the risk of being in serious danger, because in that case, it would be of the utmost importance to protect you or any other person involved."

H= Home

Whom do you live with? Have there been any recent changes in your living arrangements? What's your lifestyle like? Whom do you speak to at home about your problems?

- Screening for intra-familial violence, running away from home, a lack of supervision or financial support.

E=Education, school

Do you value your school experience? What are your motivations for going there (or not going there)? Do you have problems at school? Since when? What activities are you involved in outside of school? What are your plans for further down the road?

- Screening for regular school absenteeism, academic failures. Being careful about recent drops in academic results.

A=Activities, friends

Do you have any hobbies? What kind of activities do you do for pleasure-physical activities, activities with friends? Who are your friends? Do you have friends with whom you can share confidences? Do you work?

- Screening for isolation or social withdrawal: an absence of activities that bring about pleasure, exploitation at work.

D=Diet, nutrition

What do you eat like? What kinds of foods do you like? Do you think your nutrition is balanced? Are you happy with your body weight? Do you want to lose weight? Do you diet?

- Screening for eating disorders: desire to lose weight in spite of a normal BMI, desire to lose muscle mass, the stoppage of medications.

S= Sleep, consumption of substances, mental health issues, suicide. Your quality of sleep. Do you have problems falling asleep? Do you wake up often? Do you feel best in the morning or in the evening?

Substances: Do you consume any kind of drugs on a regular basis? (Tobacco, alcohol, drugs, medications: when started taking, frequency of use, amounts). Also, the bringing up of gambling and money problems.

Mood: Do you feel sad, down in the dumps, stressed out, anxious, or aggressive on a regular basis? Have you already thought about suicide? Have you already attempted suicide or have you talked about it?

- Screening for psychoaffective disorders, drug addiction and its consequences: school absenteeism or expulsion, conduct with weakened faculties, at-risk sexual behaviors, problems with the law. Regular problems falling asleep (depressive thoughts, substance abuse).

Early start with consumption of substances: regular or polyconsumption (disordered, depressive thoughts or the beginnings of psychosis).
Ongoing sadness (a good indicator of a depressed condition), previous suicide attempts

S=Sexuality
(Don't assume that he/she is sexually active or prejudge his/her sexual orientation).
Are you presently involved in a love relationship? Or have you ever experienced one? Do you foresee having sexual relationships in the future? Have you already had sexual relations? With a boy, a girl, or both? Did those relationships go like you wanted them to? Has it already happened that you have experienced sexual advances from others that were against your will? Do you use protection against pregnancy and STD's?

- Screening for sexual abuse, violence in love relationships, risk of pregnancy, and/or STD's.

3.3. At-Risk Behaviors: The Use of Short-Term Intervention [24]

The principles of short-term intervention are as effective with adolescents as they are with adults.

Ask the adolescent the following questions:

- How many cigarettes a day do you smoke?
- How many times a week do you drink beer and how much do you drink?
- How much do you consume when you go out or in the evenings when you are with friends?

All this is already enough to become aware of any possible problems.

Make the connection between consumption and sleep problems, chronic cough, and limited exertion…awareness of the same is still an improvement of the situation.

The effectiveness of the intervention will increase with the repetition of these questions as one continues on through the consultations.

On the other hand, paternalistic or moralistic discourse is the best way to disrupt contact with the young person and he/she will vanish into thin air.

The young person is asking for objective, not moralistic, information. Demonstrating the relationships between his/her tobacco use and the exacerbation of his/her asthma can be useful, just like showing the link between h is/her esophagitis and his/her reckless consumption of alcoholic beverages on the weekend.

Point out the mental manipulation that is occasioned by targeting through advertising. Substances induce dependence and social pressure can also be an element that induces a change, like it does with a lot of adults.

It is important to be able to play down the significance of occasional consumption but also to bear in mind that certain personality types, or certain life situations that young people may be involved in, make them at risk for dependency and/or problematic consumption. Moreover, it is helpful to say this to them.

3.3.1. Tobacco [24-25-26]

Addiction to tobacco is a major public health problem. 80-90% of adult smokers started during adolescence. More than half of adolescents who smoke are dependent on tobacco and are still smoking 5 years later.

One young person out of three is a smoker and one out of two have already smoked at least once. And among the former, 16% consume more than 16 cigarettes a day. On the other hand, 49% of all young people have never smoked while only 20% have never taken an alcoholic drink [27].

While physician intervention for weaning off tobacco is qualified as being as effective for adolescents as it is for adults, intervention does not seem to be as effective as far as the prevention of tobacco addiction is concerned.

Steady smokers are not as happy about their consumption and their dependence as they say they are. They ask for objective information. Explaining to them how strong the dependence on nicotine is and causing them to reflect on the matter is a first, indispensable step. The dependence on tobacco is strong and weaning oneself off of it is not a willpower issue. Messages about the weaning should be positive and should not emphasize failures. Encouragement should be the rule since the adolescent often suffers from very poor self-esteem.

As for the majority of smokers, but all the more for adolescent smokers, the immediate inconveniences and advantages of smoking are crucial. While from the point of view of its advantages the adolescent will mainly point out the social aspect of tobacco consumption, it is often necessary to look at the inconveniences it causes in his/her actual life: more rapid onset of dyspnea, poor sports performance, shortness of breath, all the money that has to be set aside for the cigarettes, respiratory tract infections, diminished sexual performance, etc.

As for any patient, it is pertinent to ask questions about tobacco consumption, as well as about alcohol consumption, while quantifying it every year.

The management of tobacco weaning is well-studied and documented [24-25].

The amount of help that young people derive from tobacco weaning is identical to that for adults while it is known that motivation for quitting should be looked into from the point of view of the prohibitive cost of tobacco products, the immediate undesirable effects from consumption that the young person has to become aware of, and his/her revolt against the mental and physical manipulation of which he/she is the object and is exercised upon him/her via advertising and by the product itself.

3.3.2. Alcohol

Alcohol seems to begin to take hold earlier and earlier during adolescence with a risk for chronicity that is far from negligible. This occurs, as well as an acute danger for a significant taking hold of the adolescent by alcohol at the medical (ethylic coma) or social (rolling accidents, risk-taking, unprotected sexual relations) levels. Moreover, the taking over of the young person's life by the alcohol is all the more harmful from addiction as his/her central nervous system is in the process of developing and is fully organized.

Repeated or chronic high levels of alcohol consumption interferes with cognitive processes and the structure of the personality. Therefore, the consequences could be frightening and involve the young person's medical and social prognosis.

A marked correlation has been shown between alcohol and tobacco consumption, without a doubt because of the mechanisms of addiction as well as the fact that the predisposing factors are the same for both.

Likewise, consumption of cannabis is rarely an isolated phenomenon as it is practically always related to tobacco dependency.

3.3.2.1. Just How Significant is the Problem?

A study was carried out in France at the end of 2000, within the parameters of different types of adolescent education.

A large study on young people's (ages 10-16) relationship with alcohol also took place in Belgium in 2000-2001 [29].

What were the conclusions of these studies?

The initial contact with alcohol is often made at a family party at the average age of 13. Consumption of alcohol is generally carried out among friends or when adolescents go out to nightclubs. With boys, it can also take place within the context of a sports activity: the football club refreshment room, which is a place of privilege where there is a "third half-time" after the match. The player's virility, the feeling of belonging to a group, one's thirst, and the need to relax are all intensified. This is also an at-risk location for the initial contact with alcohol for the youngest of adolescents. It is a place where this consumption is commonplace, if not glorified. However, 81% of all young people state that they do not feel pressured to drink by the group. Nevertheless, drinking with others reinforces the feeling of belonging to the group.

Adolescents consume alcohol in massive amounts, in a party frame of mind, through repeated experiences of exhilaration, mixing it with other psychoactive substances to maximize the effects. Consumption becomes more and more targeted at the consumption of hard liquor and cocktails.

The first incidence of drunkenness takes place on average at 15 ½ years of age, with no significant statistical differences between boys and girls.

Consumption of alcohol is taking place at an increasingly younger age and touches the lives of both sexes. However, for males, the precocity of the first incidence of drunkenness, and the regular consumption of tobacco and/or cannabis are clearly factors for high risk.

3.3.2.2. Screening and Assessment: The Modified CRAFFT Questionnaire [30]

Different questionnaires have been drawn up and validated for the screening of problematic alcohol consumption, one of which is FACE, which has been clearly validated by the WHO for patients who are 18 or older.

Luckily, alcohol dependence is rare during adolescence. The style of adolescent alcohol consumption is differentiated from that of adults because of its sporadic (but repetitive) and excessive party aspect.

Therefore, its abuse is essentially characterized by at-risk and harmful usage. These 2 behaviors should be screened very early to avoid the chronic evolution towards dependency.

The CRAFFT (Car, Relax, Alone, Forget, Friends/Family, Trouble) questionnaire was validated in the United States in 1998. This test has been modified since the laws are different in the United States from those in France (driver's license at 18 in France compared to 16 in the United States, commonplace moderate consumption in France for example, having one glass of wine with a meal which has no correlation to addictive behavior.)

The Modified CRAFFT Questionnaire

1. Have you ever ridden in a car that was driven by someone who had too much to drink?
2. Do you use alcohol to relax, feel better, or just to be holding onto a glass?
3. Does it so happen that you drink alcohol when you're alone?
4. Have you ever forgotten to do things you needed to after drinking alcohol?
5. Did you have any problems while you were consuming alcohol?
6. Have your family or friends said that you should cut down your consumption of alcoholic beverages?
7. Have you ever driven a 2-wheeler vehicle (bike, motorscooter, or motorbike, etc.) after having drunk too much?

The possible responses are "Often, Sometimes, Never (Often/Sometimes=1 point, Never= 1 points)

As regards alcohol consumption, the CRAFFT questionnaire is obviously shorter and more effective than tests for adults (FACS, AUDIT) because of the need to take immediate charge of the situation, with a sensitivity score of 75% and a specificity score of 76%, based on two positive responses. This test has the advantage of also being able to be adapted for and applicable to other addictive substances that require that someone take charge, such as in the case of cannabis. It also has the advantage of spotting and making the adolescent become aware of at-risk consumption, without judging or stigmatizing. Therefore, it allows for the startup of dialogue, which is often tricky.

3.3.3. Cannabis [31]

Rare are the consumers of cannabis who do not smoke something else in the first place. In France, during 2001, 60% of 19-year-old boys consumed cannabis at least once during the elapsed year. Among the 16 and 17 year-old age group, 42% of boys and 34% of girls stated that they had consumed some [32].

The major risk associated with occasional cannabis use is the risk of an accident (moped, automobile, drowning), all the more so since party consumption is rarely done in isolation and is frequently associated with tobacco use and, above all, alcohol. Only 5.5% of young people who consume have experimented with other psychoactive substances. Dependency on cannabis is weak (10%) in relation to the 30% rate for regular tobacco. The risk for intensive and frequent smoking of cannabis is dependent on multiple factors. The lack of confidence in onseself, difficulties in resolving communication problems, difficulties confronting difficult situations, consumption of tobacco and/or alcohol at an early age, personality disorders, but also the seeking out of strong sensations are some of the risk factors that arise from the consumption of psychoactive substances.

With intensive-use consumers, there are changes in short-term memory. Studies on the persistence of this effect, as well as on motivation and/academic and professional performance, are contradictory. The rate of schizophrenia is clearly higher with steady consumers of cannabis, a risk that is even higher in the case of early consumption (15% at 15 years of age). Regular consumption disturbs the menstrual cycle in young women and diminishes testosterone levels in men, causing a decrease of libido and sexual performance, which in and of itself might be a reason that would motivate someone to stop using.

Consumption should send out an alert signal to the physician when it becomes systematic to the point of having a negative effect on one's school or social life. In this case, it can be a signal of alarm if a young person is experiencing psychological suffering, but likewise, if a young person might be going off into a psychotic state on account of which he/she calms the anxiety related to the symptoms by self-medicating with cannabis [31].

The young person in front of us is asking for this kind of information. Risk-taking and notions about what is pleasurable is not the same for adolescents as it is for adults.

The use of cannabis has become commonplace. Therefore, it is necessary to speak to him/her as an adult while giving him/her facts and information about the dangers without demonizing it, but also without trivializing it. The young person needs his/her difficulties and choices understood. It is necessary to listen to them and demonstrate to him/her that the use of substances, such as they are, is hardly an effective way, and that it's even a harmful way, of resolving his/her problems.

3.3.4. The Role of the General Practitioner [33]

The general practitioner is on the front line for screening difficult consumption problems. As regards alcohol use, 90% of family doctors take over responsibility for their alcoholic patients. But in order to follow them it is imperative that the doctor think it through. But general practitioners underestimate the alcoholic consumption of the young people who consult with them. Their style of consumption being different than that of adults and the clinical presentation of the alcohol problem being even more frustrated than that of adults, the majority of doctors cannot imagine that the young person in front of them could have an alcohol problem. It is then all the more important to systematically request a quantification of this consumption. This can easily be requested during a systematic anamnesis for preventative measures (number of cigarettes smoked per day, number of colas drunk per day, number of cups of coffee per day, number of classes of (TN: Missing word) per weekend or per day, weekend, weekly, or maybe consumption of illegal substances). It is also important to be aware of what young people as well as adults expect of themselves and that they consider being questioned about this matter legitimate.

64% of tobacco smokers are identified as such by their doctors. On the other hand, only 15% of young people who have been intoxicated at least once have been found out.

Likewise, 35.7% of occasional cannabis users have been screened while regular users are not. This is surprising because while 11 general practitioners out of 13 do not approach the problem of alcohol with their young patients, they are aware that there is a family history of alcohol use with 16% of the young people who came for a consultation. Why is this so? Perhaps it is because the doctors, who have often been the family physician since the patient's early childhood in 52% of the cases, does not perceive that the young person before him is turning into an adult and can have some adult behaviors, including those of addiction. Moreover, the image of alcohol in our society is extremely ambiguous. Alcohol is not only a possible health problem, but also a social problem.

In effect, there is an obvious lack of information for doctors concerning the addictive behaviors of young people, above all, with regard to alcohol. This is why it is important that doctors make use of the tools in existence, not only systematic anamnesis that is concerned with all behaviors of consumption, but also standardized questionnaires such as the modified CRAFFT.

4. Unhappiness, Depression, and Suicide [34]

Depression is a significant problem during adolescence, the consequences of which can be dramatic. It is likewise an under-diagnosed problem, whether it be because the physician doesn't investigate the situation during a consultation or because the young person is more willing to talk about it with friends and will not seek out a spontaneous consultation for that. He/she will eventually be brought in for a consultation by his/her parents or a friend.

Between 1989 and 1991, the suicide rate in Brussels (Belgium) for young people ages 15-24 rose to 12/100,000 with a sex ratio of 4 to 1 in favor of young men (whose rate is 19/100,000). This means that in Brussels, 1 adolescent out of every 8,000 will commit suicide. Generally speaking, one has to consider that a young person who has attempted suicide carries 20x the risk of trying it again over a young person with no previous history of attempts. 10% of suicide attempts are followed by a repeat attempt within the following 3 months.

In industrialized countries, suicide is the second leading cause of death for males ages 15 through 25, after accidents, and the third leading cause for young women, after cancer ailments. Between the ages of 12 and 19, 2 or 3 young people out of 10 say that they have had suicidal thoughts and among those, 8 , that is to say a little less than 1 adolescent out of 10, have gone on to the act.

And what is frightening is that the majority of them, even those who have been hospitalized, have not had any help or follow-up whatsoever…And it just so happens that people not taking the underlying feelings or distress into account is a major factor in the subsequent attempt; in this case, 1 out of 3 young people try again within 6 months with a heightened lethal risk.

The psychopathological consequences in the adult years are far from insignificant and therefore, the possibility of another suicide attempt cannot be trivialized.

4.1. Obstacles to Screening and Prevention

There are two main reasons why primary prevention is difficult:

1. The young person does not talk to the referring adults about his/her problems. He/she has an instinctive mistrust of adults who "do not understand." He/she is more willing to talk to peers about it who will sometimes bring him/her in for a consultation.

Although 2 out of 3 adolescents speak to their friends about their suicidal thoughts, only 1 out of 5 speak to their parents about it. When there is a suicide attempt, only 1 out of 2 adolescents has spoken about it to a friend (in 75% of the cases), and more rarely to a parent (1 out of 10).

2. Moreover, adults in general, and above all parents, have significant difficulties seeing and recognizing the preliminary signs of morbid ideation in what they see as their children's simple, generalized feelings of unhappiness. Their problems are trivialized and minimized. The low death rate for first attempts (8 to 16% survive) engenders a trivialization of suicide attempts. One musn't ignore the fact either that the suicidal thoughts of their children give parents feelings of powerlessness and failure that is difficult for them to accept.
3. The acting out of the suicidal act is not always premeditated, even if it takes place at a place that is predisposed to it. 55% of suicidal adolescents confirm they hadn't premeditated about it at all, 71% did not warn anyone they were going to do it, and 76% did not carry out any preparations.

Astonishingly, in secondary prevention, the great majority of parents do not know that their child has made a suicidal gesture. Moreover, there still is a feeling that one needs to trivialize the suicidal gesture, above all if there are no somatic consequences to the act. One is more willing to talk about a young person who has taken psychiatric medications than a suicidal young person. But the risk for repeating the attempt has no relation to the somatic seriousness of the first attempt. Moreover, if one takes into account the underlying distress, it is not always easy to take charge of it in view of the lack of specialized facilities. On average, 1 out of 10 suicidal adolescents will have a consultation with a regular health professional, whereas a lower proportion will meet with a psychologist or psychiatrist.

4.2. The Ambiguity of the Family Physician's Role

Although the doctor's familiarity with the family can be an advantage on account of the reciprocal confidence created throughout the course of their years working together and because of the doctor's knowledge of family problems, it can also be a handicap.

Indeed, because of shame or pride, the adolescent's difficulties, associated with a feeling of failure to educate on the part of the parents, might be hidden. Moreover, rightly or wrongly, certain family members might think that the doctor is showing partiality.

4.3. Screening of Unhappy Adolescents

In a generalist medical practice, to be called upon for an adolescent suicide problem is very rare: it occurs less than once per year [36]. Less than 10% of persons with suicidal tendencies talk to their doctor about it beforehand [37]. On the other hand these crisis situations have often been preceded by warning symptoms [38]. And 30% of adolescents are affected by depressive episodes [39]. The adolescent is characterized by an emotionalism that is often exacerbated by a significant reactivity to events [40]. A breakup of a love relationship can therefore trigger a depressive scenario.

Therefore, it is necessary to be aware that the "major depression" of an adolescent groups together 3 medical entities:

- Adjustment problems
- Major unipolar depression
- Bipolar depression

It is often difficult to make a distinction between an adjustment problem, a feeling of sadness following a specific event, and an actual depression. This explains the spontaneous recovery, after a few days, of some young people who have been labeled as having major depression.

In addition, major depression in nearly half of the adolescents evolves into bipolar depression (manic-depression).

Symptoms Causing Unipolar Depression	Symptoms Causing Manic Episodes
Change in mood (irritability, sadness)	Change in mood (irritability, exaltation)
Loss of self-esteem, self destructive behaviors, self-mutilation	Increase in self-esteem and/or ideas of grandeur
Sleep disorders (insomnia, hyersomnia)	Reduction in the need to sleep
Trouble concentrating, difficulties in making decisions.	Distraction, flight of ideas
Anhedonia and lack of interest	Excessive engagement in pleasurable activities that are potentially dangerous
Fatigue	
Ruminations +/- suicidal	Logorrhea, chattering
Psychomotor slackening or agitation	Psychomotor agitation or increase in directed activities (social, sexual, school)

At the time of the initial consultation, it is practically impossible to make a clean-cut diagnosis, even for a psychiatrist. This means that it is necessary for the general physician to take care to maximize as much as possible his/her sensitivity, starting with the first consultation, not only to facilitate a quick start at taking charge of the situation as optimally as possible, but also to allow for the establishment of an atmosphere of trust, such that the young person will feel that he/she has been listened to and so that he/she will return. Indeed, the time spent with the general practitioner, who is a valuable ally, will progressively allow him/her to make an exact diagnosis of the problem.

Therefore, it is important to be able to screen for this problem and correctly and easily take charge of it in a systematic way. It just so happens that all the current referentials are adapted to the management of crisis situations which will necessitate a transfer over to a specialized service.

Few studies attempted to create a standardized screening method in relation to a behavior that was to subsequently take place.

A French consensus conference, under the aegis of the ANAES (Agence Nationale de l'Acreditation et d'Évaluation en Santé, TN: National Agency for Health Accreditation and Assessment), which dealt with the crisis of suicide issued some proposals so that the general practitioner would be able to utilize special tools specifically adapted for daily consultations to help him/her reach decisions in his/her practice [41].

Starting from the principle that suicidal thoughts are not systematic with every adolescent and that suicidal antecedents are a risk factor for moving on again to a suicidal act, and that bringing up this problem with the young person does not favor him/her for going ahead with the act [42], a group of general practitioners and French psychiatrists from the cities have, along with this consensus, created and experimented with a practice/approach test for the screening of suicidal tendencies.

4.3.1. The Consultation Referential for the General Practitioner [43]

It strives towards 2 goals:

1. To broaden the scope of consultation
2. And, in the event there is a problem, to help the adolescent move beyond this hurdle.

It is supported by 4 basic attitudes:

1. To make conditions for patient expression favorable by laying out a time for talking
2. To create a therapeutic atmosphere by making conditions favorable for the adolescents comfort and feelings of security in which he/she achieves autonomy.
3. To improve the patient's capacity for self-acceptance and the accurate representation of his/her body image in order to create conditions conducive to good self-esteem.
4. To give rise to a diversity of possible solutions from which the patient will choose.

The HEADS Questionnaire has already been mentioned. It allows the practitioner to formulate an idea of the young person's psychosocial experience and enables him/her to carry out a screening beforehand for risk factors and possible problems that might require assistance.

All the physician's art will consist of understanding the young person's complaint and of flushing out the possible real reasons for the consultation. In the first place, it will sometimes be a matter of making conditions favorable for dialogue with the patient leaving him/her with more freedom to speak and act, among other things by asking those that have accompanied him/her to leave him alone with the young person.

It is sometimes necessary to clarify the situation by asking who has actually requested the consultation and for what reason. But there must also be agreement regarding what can be said, the reason for it to be spoken, and how and why it is to be said.

It is likewise necessary to open doors by attempting to go beyond the symptom or the complaint that was brought into the consultation, for example, by asking, "Is there anything else you would like to talk to me about or that is on your mind?"

In the event that a problem is revealed, it is important to:

1. Reformulate the complaint and the expression of the same.
2. Reinforce the doctor-patient bond so that the adolescent feels safe.
3. Fix a time for a meeting inside of a deadline that is proportional to the young person's distress.
4. Direct the patient to a specialized facility if necessary.

4.3.2. The TSTS – CAFARD Test: Screening for Suicidal Tendencies [43-44-45]

It consists of a 4-themed approach by asking open-ended questions.

These 4 themes are: Traumatology, Sleep, Tobacco Use, Stress (T.S.T.S.)

For each positive response, there is a corresponding question that is introduced according to its degree of seriousness, which includes 5 key words: Nightmares, Aggressive Behaviors, Daily Incidence of Smoking, Absenteeism, Disagreeable Experience in Relation to Family (C.A.F.A.R.D.S.).

1 out of 2 adolescent with suicidal ideation gives two positive responses to at least two different questions.

Themes T.S.T.S	Open-Ended Question	Level of Seriousness for Evaluation if Positive C.A.F.A.R.D.	Corresponding Question
Traumatology	Experienced trauma within the last 12 months?	Aggressive Behaviors	Have you been a victim of aggression?
Sleep	Difficulty with falling asleep or frequently awake?	Nightmares	Are there recurring themes?
Tobacco Use	Active or former smoker?	Active smoker	Do you smoke every day? Is it associated with other consumptions? (Cannabis or alcohol)
Stress	Feeling of tension, stress, anxiety related to school and/or a family problem	Stress at school: Absenteeism	Frequent school absences or tardiness?
		Family stress: disagreeable family experience	Feeling of insecurity, discomfort, malaise within the family

4.4. Depression and Suicide

Adolescent suicide does not always arise from an underlying depressive condition: depression is found only 40% of suicidal patients. Moreover, adolescent depression is definitely masked by complaints or behaviors about which questions must be asked.

On the other hand, there is a quasi-systematic feeling of failure and a devaluation of oneself. Somatization of anxiety occurs frequently and is a reason for which these young people seek out a consultation. A suicidal gesture, moreover, could come about from a panic attack.

4.4.1. Traps and Difficulties [46]

Several factors are in opposition to the family doctor taking responsibility for young people who are suffering:

1. The family doctor is often far removed from and barely familiar with the social and psychological care networks.
2. Being in a direct battle with the young person and his/her family, he has trouble putting up a resistance to the family's trivializing discourse, which is a consequence of the young person's very own denial.
3. The significant difficulty in finding help or support while the situation is going on induces a significant amount of discouragement.

If the doctor's attitude validates the trivialization of the problem, this is a major factor in his/her not taking charge, and consequently, it is a factor for a poor prognosis, with an increased risk of death.

The literature, however, demonstrates the importance, on the level of prognosis, of the psychiatric and systematic take-over of any suicidal person's case. And all the more so since this taking over of responsibility is carried out by a therapist who specializes in adolescent psychopathology. This thorough taking over of responsibility is accomplished with the cooperation of the young person and his/her family.

4.4.2. Alarm Signals [46]

Although young people go for a consultation with their family doctor for psychological problems rather infrequently (1 in 13 adolescents), 1 in 9 who have suicidal ideation consult for that reason, and 1 in 5 have gone on to the act.

Moreover, consultations because of various physical complaints, mainly fatigue and headaches, markedly increase with young people who experience suicidal ideation and the same continues to increase within the 6 months prior to going ahead with the act. Also, requests for disability certificates, school absenteeism, but also overconsumption of medications for various problems (headaches, backaches, nervousness, insomnia, etc.) are, just as much, signals for help.

This means that any consultation with an adolescent is a chance to not fail to engage in dialogue with the adolescent and go further.

4.4.3. The at-Risk Population [46]

According to the Canadian study group's recommendations for preventative health care, [47], evaluation of suicide risk is recommended when the patient is part of an at-risk group. If a diagnosis of depression is present, medical treatment is recommended.

What are the adolescent risk factors for suicide?

- A family history of psychiatric illness
- Depression
- Drug and alcohol abuse, especially if the patient is isolated.
- Terminal phase chronic illness
- Ethnic minority adolescent males
- Family history of suicide
- First-generation immigrant women

The treating physician will be all the more attentive if the young person:

1. Presents with problems related to school (failure, absenteeism, etc). There is a marked statistical correlation between failure, disengagement, flight from situations, and suicidal behaviors.
2. Demonstrates behavior disorders (agressivity, stealing, isolating him/herself, etc.)
3. Presents with recurring somatic complaints headaches, lumbago, fatigue, stomach aches, sleep disorders, etc.
4. Is a member of a family in crisis or in which there is no communication: divorce, discord, chronic conflicts, violence, psychological disorders in one or both parents, failed parenting, etc.
5. Or conversely, in a family where the bonds between the suicidal adolescent and his/her family are too intense. This means that any event, even if it seems to be trivial, can be experienced as an abandonment or rejection, impelling one on to the suicidal act.

It will likewise be a matter of assessing:

1. The quality of familial bonds as well as the family histories of psychiatric illness or suicide. Denial of difficulties by the parents, as a case in point, is an indication of their seriousness.
2. The quality of friendship bonds. It is a matter of evaluating if the network to which the patient belongs offers him/her positive social supports.
3. Integration into school life and the existence of some self-actualization at this level. This is also a positive aspect.
4. The adolescent's relationship with his/her body. If it is harmonious, it has to do with being a balancing factor.
5. Antecedents of intra- or extrafamilial violence or sexual abuse. These are pejorative elements.
6. Drug consumption. If it is a regular and, above all, solitary activity, it cannot be trivialized, just as in the case of excessive and repeated alcohol consumption.
7. Impulsive, aggressive, and explosive behaviors. This could quickly lead to suicidal behavior.

4.4.4. Lethal Risk Factors Based on a Suicide Attempt [6]

There is no strict relationship between the significance of the desire for death and the lesions associated with a suicide attempt. On the other hand, the violence associated with the attempt is often a pejorative indicator. 4 somatic risk factors have been identified:

- Social isolation
- Intrafamilial problems
- Family history of sexual abuse: rapes and incest have occurred 2x as frequently in cases where there has been a suicide attempt.
- Psychiatric disorders: 90% of young people of lethal risk have a psychiatric diagnosis. Therefore, these patients make up a high risk group. This might cause one to consider that not sending a young suicidal person to a psychiatrist whose clinical specialty is adolescent behavior is a medical mistake.

4.4.5. The Physician's Attitude when Confronted with a Suicide Attempt or the Risk of the Same [46]

4.4.5.1. The Bringing up of Depressive Thoughts

As was already stated above, it is important for the young person to understand that his unhappiness has been listened to and has been seriously thought through. In addition, the physician should clearly demonstrate that he/she is ready and capable of making his/her way with the patient as a reaction against the latter's anxieties about death, without dramatizing, but neither minimizing them.

It then is necessary to investigate through dialogue what it is that brings up the depressive thoughts that pass through the patient's mind, which are possibly secondary to a specific event, or because of a well-constructed suicide plan.

The exploration of the patient's internal world (feelings, personal obstacles, etc.) and the world outside of him/herself, will then allow him/her to engage in dialogue about possible solutions. On the other hand, if the despair, the feeling that there is not way out, and violence and rage are forcefully expressed, the physician should express his/her real anxiety and his/her desire to protect the patient. This requires regular follow-ups that are coordinated with the doctor's availability, something that should be clearly stated to the patient. This will also require psychotherapeutic follow-up, individual or family, with or without combined drug therapy. This obviously immediately poses the problem of the costs involved: the anti-depressant medication is reimbursed but the psychotherapy is not, something that really makes it impossible for adolescents and for many families. The orientation towards mental health or family planning centers can resolve the issue of the cost, in part, while being aware that delays in having one's case taken on at such places can be long.

4.4.5.2. Recognized Suicide Attempts

Any act of aggression towards oneself is considered a suicide attempt, whatever methods are implemented, along with their resulting morbidity. This is so even if the wish to die is not explicit.

It is important for the physician to welcome the adolescent patient and listen to his/her distress, even if the latter goes through an emergency service, for he/she will only very rarely have been seen and listened to by a psychologist or a psychiatrist. The parents involved should also be welcomed and listened to. This will allow the physician to make a precise evaluation and solidly engage the parents and the young person in starting up with a specialized psychotherapeutic monitoring program. To organize the practice modalities, they will be seen together so that any misunderstandings or manipulation will be avoided. In the event of a clear refusal of treatment on the part of the family or young person, or if there is a high risk that there will be a repeated attempt with a significant lethal risk, the possibility of hospitalization in a specialized setting should be brought up, possibly against the patient's will, within the framework of the law that has to do with the protection of the mentally ill. This is rare and is mainly to be found within the context of obvious psychiatric disorders that involve a high risk of suicide and a refusal by or an inability of the family to keep up with regular follow-ups.

5. Adolescent Self-Esteem, Love Relationships and Sexuality

Having one's first experience of a totally fulfilling love relationship is not a simple thing. The affirmation of the self, which is associated to respect from the other, the awareness of one's limits and those of the other person involved, the respecting of or non-respecting of these limits, and the personal values that guide one's life are problems to be resolved so that one can develop his/her personality. It just so happens, as the Ottawa Charter [48] states, that "good mental health also comes about from the ability to make decisions and control the conditions of one's life."

The best definition of the affirmation of the self seems to be that of Ginette Larouche [49]: "The affirmation of the self resides in refusing to be passive and refusing to forget about oneself, things that are encouraged by stereotypes. The person who affirms him/herself gives enough value to his/her life so that they have power over it. He/she expresses his/her emotions, needs, and rights in a sustained fashion and based on the respect from the other."

It is of major importance for the young person to be able to affirm him/herself and to have enough confidence in him/herself. Indeed, not only is it his/her well-being that is optimized, but also his/her capacity for success. But besides, this will allow him/her to improve his/her capacity for building stable emotional and loving relationships. In effect, it is the best way to prevent violence between partners, but also, any kind of interpersonal violence.

5.1. Love and Sexual Relationships: The State of the Issue

In the French-speaking community of Belgium, the Socialist Provident Women's Federation of Family Planning (Fédération des Centres de Planning Familial des Femmes Prévoyantes Socialistes) conducted a study with 13 to 21 year-olds from November of 2005 through January of 2006. There were 650 respondents [50]. This study is discussed in great detail here because it has quite recently created a very interesting picture of this problem.

Two age categories were designed: the 13-16 year-olds (the "young group"), and the 16-21 year-olds (the "older group").

It is necessary to note right away that the young group sometimes had trouble differentiating between all the various types of sexual experiences which necessitated questions that were more precise.

As for the responses to the question regarding their knowledge of what is important for them in a couple's relationship, respect for and trust in the other are practically equal (at 30% each), coming out ahead of sexuality (23%). Although trust is the most important value for both girls and boys, respect is the value most advanced by girls (58%) as opposed to 29% for boys. Conversely, sexuality is the most important for boys (43%) as opposed to 18% for girls.

59.9% of all young people (61% of girls and 58.3% of boys) who were questioned have already had a sexual relationship. If one analyzes the results as a function of age, 48.8% of the youngest (<16 years old) and 78.2% of the oldest have already had a complete sexual relationship. The average age of the first sexual experience is 15, and that is as true for girls as it is for boys.

An important fact is that 7.3% of young people have had a sexual experience somewhere between 4 and 12 y ears of age.

The obvious rape or incest hypothesis is, unfortunately, involved here. This is an element that the physician should be very much on the lookout for.

If one differentiates the young people as a function of the type of education pursued, it is interesting to note that 64.6% of the young people coming out of a technical education, and 60.9 coming out of a professional education have had a sexual relationship. This is compared to 42.4% of young people with a general education who state that they have already had one.

It should be noted, just the same, that 10% of the young people questioned (8.1% of boys and 11.1% of girls) have not yet had sexual experience of any type (flirting, petting, intercourse, etc.)

5.1.1. Motivation for the First Sexual Experience

The responses vary, according to sex.

The first reason put forward is obviously feelings of love. It was recognized as the reason by 75.4% of girls and 59.5% of boys. On the other hand, they indicate sexual desire in practically equal numbers, with 51% for boys versus 35.5% for girls. Girls brought up other reasons: sexual curiosity, the request for sex by her partner, even if he had no personal desire for it, the desire to lose her virginity and feel like an adult, or to be doing what everyone else is doing. This last reason, as well as sexual curiosity, are more of a motivation for boys. On the other hand, in 2.3% of cases, the girls felt forced to do it. Therefore, it would seem that social pressure, and/or pressure from one's partner is far from being a negligible factor in this regard, and above all, as far as boys are concerned.

5.1.2. Homosexual Versus Heterosexual

4.6% mention a first homosexual experience. Girls mention one in 6.7% of cases as opposed to boys who only mention one in 1.3% of the cases.

5.1.3. Their Partners

49.6% have had several sexual encounters with the same partner and 42.1% with multiple partners. Girls mentioned having just one partner more often, in contradistinction to boys.

A surprising fact is that 49.7% of students with a technical education have had multiple partners as opposed to 35% of students with a professional education and 29.8% with a general education. With the last two educational groups, sexual relations are more often with just one partner (57.4% for the general education group and 56% for the professional education group).

5.1.4. Self Affirmation in Love Relationships

This issue was extensively investigated in the study with different questions:

- Going out with a girl/boy without feeling obligated to have sexual relations with him/her.

78.6% of girls don't see any problem in this. On the other hand, 23.23% of boys feel obligated to have sexual intercourse. Conversely, 6.92% of girls feel they are confronted with strong pressure because of their partner's demand for it as opposed to 5.51% of boys. The majority of young people, independent of age, feel they are capable of determining the moment when they are ready to have sexual relations, but this is only true for a preponderance of girls.

- Refusal to participate in a sexual practice that the young person does not feel comfortable with.

By a substantial majority, the girls again respond that they would easily refuse. On the other hand, for 55.9% of the boys, this reasoning is more difficult. As one's age increases, self-affirmation becomes more marked. The type of education is likewise an important factor: young people with general or technical education find it easier to refuse.

- Communication at the level of desire.

56% of young people have difficulties communicating about what would increase their sexual pleasure. Less than 1 out of every 2 girls dare to talk to their partner about what would increase their pleasure as opposed to almost 3 out of 4 boys who clearly state what it is that would give them pleasure.

- Attitudes Toward Contraception

12% of young people admit that they don't know if their partner had picked up any means of contraception at the time of their first experience of sexual intercourse! 1 boy in 5 doesn't know if his partner uses any kind of birth control!

Among the contraceptive methods used the first time a young person has sexual intercourse, 1 out of 2 of them used a condom, 1 out of 10 use birth control pills only, and 1 out of 5 used a condom along with birth control pills. This is the only way to protect oneself against pregnancy and sexually transmitted diseases. In spite of everything, 15% of young people still didn't use protection the first time they had intercourse. But conversely, 85% of young people used protection afterwards, something that is very encouraging and reassuring.

4 out of 5 young people state that they can easily get a hold of some form of contraception. This obviously seems to be all the more true as the young person advances in age.

Talking about contraception with one's partner does not always seem to be the easiest thing to do, especially for girls, all the more so when they are a younger age. When all ages and both sexes are mixed together, 6% of young people do not talk about contraception with their partner before they have sexual intercourse.

On the other hand, girls are clearly more comfortable with refusing to have intercourse if they don't have the contraceptive method of their choice at their disposal (70%). This compares to 1 out of 2 boys who would have problems refusing. Again, refusal seems to be all the more easier for a young person who attends general or technical school as opposed to one who attends a professional school.

In conclusion, even so, it is noteworthy that the majority of young people know how to impose limits in the area of sexual relations regarding their choice of partner, when they will have sexual relations, and about the use of contraception. But on the whole, this seems to be more difficult for boys, the youngest of adolescents, and students who are in professional schools.

5.2. The Role of the Family Doctor [6]

In view of the preceding, the general practitioner's role, whether he/she is a traditional family doctor chosen by the adolescent or a family planning doctor, is important for setting up guidelines for young people. When young people ask for contraception, or simply at the time of a routine visit or checkup with no adult present, the doctor should be able to talk about imposing limits and about being aware of and respecting one's own desires.

Family doctors should be encouraged to support the following initiatives:

- Promote the adolescent's sexual health in accordance with the young person's sexual orientation.
- Encourage the young person to adopt responsible sexual behaviors, both at the level of pregnancy prevention and the prevention of sexually transmitted diseases. The 2 P's (in French, TN: Condoms and Birth Control Pills) and the 2 C's Rule (in English, Condoms and Contraception) should be advocated.
- Help the young person to be able to affirm and have his/her limits respected.
- Encourage parents to become aware and accept that sexuality is part of their adolescent's normal development. In effect, there are still too many teenage pregnancies associated with parents' refusal to allow them to get contraceptives, although young people can get contraception without their parents' knowledge. And besides, it is practically free in Belgium after one reaches the age of 21. The doctor should be encouraged to take the following initiatives:
- Encourage families to become involved in their children's emotional and sexual education.
- Increase young people's awareness about the problem of violence with the wrong kind of people.
- Be on the lookout so that he/she can detect victims of sexual abuse in view of the disturbing amount of sexual encounters that take place between 4 and 12 years of age which are assumed to be prosecutable.

6. Conclusion

The general practitioner is on the front line in relation to the problems of the adolescent population. Although the greatest majority of adolescents are all right in spite of having some conflicts, emotional upsets, and cases of the blues, it is important to not only screen young people who are in danger but also to prevent at-risk situations ahead of time.

Education is, in the first place, a verbal exchange and the putting in place of behavioral norms and markers. This is essentially the role of the parents and the school but also that of the doctor. The doctor has no authority over the young person like the parents and the school do, on the contrary his/her role is characterized by its informational aspect and its screening procedures. Moreover, when one speaks about a verbal exchange, that also means that not only do adults educate their adolescents, but the inverse is also true. Sometimes, the parents, as well as the doctor, should change their attitude towards the young person they are concerned about. Because in spite of the tools the physician has at his/her disposal, it is above all the way that he looks at the young person that should change.

7. References

[1] Rochefort L., Garneau L., Paquin L. L'éthique dans la pratique auprès des adolescents *Le Médecin du Québec Janvier*. 2005; 40: 49-57.

[2] Rieve AK, Di Fulvio A, Di Marco S, Volpone D (Italy) Telling stories rather than making diagnoses: a one year experience with teenage psychic discomfort in GP. An opportunity to prevent medicalization? 12th Regional conference of WONCA Europe 2006.

[3] Paulus D., Pestiaux D., Doumenc M. Teenagers and their family practitioner: matching between their reasons for encounter Family Practice 2004; 21:143-145.

[4] Office of National Statistics Death by age, sex and underlying cause in England and Wales 2003 London: Stationnery Office 2004.

[5] Department of Health Health survey for England 2002 London: stationery Office 2003.

[6] Lambert D. La prévention chez l'adolescent: comment l'aborder? *Le Médecin du Québec.* vol 40 mai 2005: 5:55-62.

[7] De la graine à l'arbre: pas facile d'être jeune Rapport du Groupe de travail sur la santé des adolescents, College des médecins de famille du Canada (MFC).

[8] McPharson A. ABC of adolescence: Adolescents in primary care, *BMJ.* 2005; 300:465-7.

[9] Oppong-Odiseng AC, Heycock EG Adolescent health services through their eyes. *Arch. Dis. Child.* 1997; 77:115-119.

[10] Cheng TL, Savageau JA, Sattler AL, Dewitt TG. Confidentiality in health care: a survey of knowledge, perceptions and attitudes among high school students. *J. Am. Med. Assoc.* 1997; 269:1404-7.

[11] Walthery C., Vandoome C., Boden CS Motivations et apports d'une prise en charge ambulatoire pluridisciplinaire de la santé des adolescents bulletin d'Éducation du patient. 2000 19(3): 126-9.

[12] Stoverinck M.-J., Lagro Janssen A.-L., Wefe C.-V. Sex differences in health problems, diagnostic testing and primary care. *J. Fam. Pract.* 1996 43 (6): 567-6.

[13] Marks A, Malizio J. Hoch 3, Brody R, Fisher M. Assessment of health needs and willingness to utilize health care resources of adolescents in a suburban population. *J. Pediatr.* 1983; 102: 456-60.

[14] Ziv A, Boulet JR, Slap GB. Utilization of physician offices by adolescents in the United States. *Pediatrics.* 1999 10:35-42.

[15] World Health Organization. Health and Health Behaviour Among Young People. *WHO Policy Séries: Health Policy for Children and Adolescents,* Issue no. 1:2000.

[16] Vers la santé des jeunes en l'an 2000? Une étude des comportements et modes de vie des adolescents de la communauté française de Belgique de 1986 à 1994 École de Santé Publique ULB Bruxelles 1997, 68p.

[17] Chambonet J.-Y., Ahssaini C., Senand R. Qu'attend du généraliste la deuxieme génération issue de l'immigration ? Une enquête réalisée à Nantes auprès d'adolescents issus de l'immigration maghrebine. *Rev Med Gen* 2000; 14(485); 145-50.

[18] Adapté de: Age-specific Charts, Ages 11-24 Years, de US Preventive Services Task Force (1996 et mises a jours) en tenant compte des recommendations canadiennes (tableau tiré de la référence suivante)

[19] Group d'étude canadien sur les soins de santé preventives, la société canadienne de pediatrie, US Preventive Services Task Force, American Medical Association, American Academy of Family Physicians, American Academy of pediatrics.

[20] Schütz C., Vaudaux B. La Vaccination à l'adolescence: rôle des praticiens et des services de santé scolaire *Revue Médicale Suisse* 2006: 69: 1522-5.

[21] van Lierde S. Vaccinations Hepatite B in *Pediatrie Capita Selecta:* 174-175 Ed. Garant 1996.

[22] Lambert D. La prévention chez l'adolescent: comment l'aborder ? *Le Médecin du Québec.* vol 40 mai 2005: 5:55-62.

[23] Association des médecins omnipraticiens de Montreal L'examen médical preventif chez les adolescents: Intervenir selon leur profil de risque Prévention en pratique médicale Québec février 2005.

[24] Gestion du sevrage tabagique FARES novembre 2003 *http://www.fares.be/documents/ArgumentaireCiScient.pdf.*

[25] Tremblay M. Interventions et outils pour les jeunes fumeurs, Institut National de Santé publique du Québec novembre 2005 *http://www.inspq.qc.ca/jasp/archives/pdf/2005/JASP2005-AbandonTabac-Tremblay1.pdf.*

[26] Laperche J., Destexhe G. and coll. Tabac et cannabis chez l'adolescent *Revue de la Médecine Générale* 2003; 208:490-495.

[27] Institut de Santé Publique, Enquête de Santé par Interviews auprès de 12000 belges en 2001.

[28] Picard V., Gerbaud L. and coll. Étude de la consummation d'alcool en milieu scolaire (l'alcool chez les adolescents II) *Rev. Prat. Med. Gen.* 2002; 16: 743-7.

[29] Santé en Hainaut Carnet de bord de la santé 2004, n 5 Observatoire de la Santé du Hainaut *http://www.hainaut.be/sane/observatoiresante/publications/medias/Carnet-de-Bord-2004.pdf.*

[30] Picard V., Gerbaud L. Validation d'un test de dépistage de l'usage nocif d'alcool (L'alcool chez les adolescents l) *Rev. Prat. Med. Gen.* 2002: 16: 699-703.

[31] Nauy J.-Y.Nouvelles lumiéres sur la noclvité du cannabis M and H 2002: 2489-1489.

[32] Etiemble J. Cannabis: quels effets sur le comportement et la santé ? *INSERM* novembre 2001.

[33] Picard V., Gerbaud L. Place du médecin de famille dans la prévention des conduits d'alcoolisation chez les adolescents (L'alcool chez les adolescents III) *Rev. Prat. Med. Gen.* 2002: 16:796-9.

[34] Association pour le dévelopment des traitements, de la prévention, de la formation et de la recherche en Santé Mentale a l'ULB Recherche Action pour une prevention du

suicide dans d'adolescence en milieu scolaire en région de Bruxelles-capitale rapport d'activité 1/12/2000-31/11/2002 *http://www.ulb.ac.be/assoc/ssm/suicid %2002.pdf.*

[35] Choquet M., Davidson F. Famille et suicide: quelle famille pour les suidants ? *Psychol. Med.* (1984); 16:2035-7.

[36] URML. Enquête sur la prise en charge des suicides et des tentatives de suicide en médicine liberale dans la region Poitou-Charente: 1997-1999.

[37] Rey C., Michaud P.A., Narring F., Perron C. Les conduits suicidaries chez les adolescents en Suisse: le rôle des médecins. *Arch. Pediatr.* 1997; 4:784-92.

[38] Links P.S. Balchand K., Dawe I, Watson WJ. Preventing recurrent suicidal behavior. *Can. Fam. Physician.* 1999; 45:265 and -60.

[39] Alvin P, Marcelli D. Médecine de l'adolescent Paris: Masson; 2005. p.151.

[40] Maranda Fr. L'omnipraticien at les troubles de l'humeur à l'adolescence Le Médecin du Québec août 2003: 38: 55-60.

[41] ANAES. *La crise suicidaire: reconnaître et prendre en charge.* Conférence de concensus. PARIS; 19-20 octobre 2000.

[42] Gould M.S., Marrocco F.A., et al. Evaluating iatrogenic risk of youth suicide screening programs: a randomized control trial. *JAMA.* 2005: 293 : 1635-43.

[43] Binder Ph., Chabaud Fr. Accueil des adolescents en médecine générale: validation de l'usage d'un réferential. *Rev. Prat. Médecine Générale.* 2005 ;710-711: 1307-13.

[44] Binder Ph. Dépister les conduits suicidaires des adolescents: conception d'un test et validation de son usage. *Rev. Prat. Med. Gen.* 2004:18 :576-80.

[45] Audit clinique auprès de 40 généralistes. *Rev. Prat. Med. Gen.* 2004; 18:641-5.

[46] Prevenir le suicide a l'adolescence: 10 questions aux généralistes sur le suicide a l'adolescence Fond Houtman Bruxelles http://www.ulb.ac.be/assoc/ssm/suicide.pdf.

[47] Groupe d'étude canadien sur les soins de santé préventifs. Canadian Task Force on Preventive Health Care: Prevention of Suicide. 1991.

[48] Charte d'Ottawa, OMS 1986 http://www.euro.who.int/AboutWHO/Policy/20010827_2?language=French.

[49] Larouche G. Tolérance Zéro Femmes et santé Ed. Fedération des infirmières et infirmiers du Québec; Québec 1997.

[50] L'affirmation de soi dans les relations amoureuses et affectives chez les jeunes: enquête menée auprès des 13-21 ans par la Fédération des Centres de Planning Familial des Femmes Prévoyantes Socialistes Mars 2006.

In: The Adolescent Today in Medicine
Editors: N. Zdanowicz, et al. pp. 125-142
ISBN: 978-1-60021-764-7

Chapter 8

Generation Cannabis: Drugs and Adolescence

P. Schepens[*1] *and K.de Marneffe*[2]

[1] Psychiatrist, Head of psychiatric unit, clinique-saint-Pierre Ottignies
[2] Post-graduate in psychiatry, Université Catholique de Louvain, Belgium

Abstract

An especially sad paradox concerns adolescents' drug use. In terms of heath consequences, adolescence is indeed the period in life during wich one is most exposed to at risk behaviors, and particularly toxic substances use. Adolescence is unfortunately also the period during which the brain, and therefore the integrity of the emotional, cognitive and relational systems is the most fragile and vulnerable. One cannot assess the impact of drug consumption on adolescents' health without taking into account this paradox and this specific vulnerability. The present chapter will attempt to reveal the knowledge we have about addictions by focusing on specific issues which link adolescence, drugs, ans public health. We will attempt to accomplish this task without falling into the trap of demagogy and taboos.

What adolescents ? What products ? What environment ? How does it work ? What is going on in the brain ? These will be the very first questions we will address. The following issues will address the personal, relational and social consequences of drug consumption, and the real nature of the risk young consumers incur. However, we cannot address those issues without first asking ourselves the crucial questions pertaining to, the meaning of adolescents' drug consumption ans how it challenges us as adults in terms of the trans generational link that ties us to adolescents. Finally, we will raise the fundamental questions that preoccupy any adult in charge of an adolescent : when should we begin worrying ? What to do ? What strategies should we implement in terms of information, prevention, risk reduction ans healthcare ?

* Contact: Clinique Saint-Pierre, avenue Reine Fabiola, 9 à 1340 Ottignies(Belgium) Tél : 003210/437.263, 003210/437.128, Fax : 003210/437.127, E.mail : pi.schepens@clinique-saint-pierre.be

Keywords: adolescence, family, health, recreational drugs, cannabis, prevention, healthcare, hyper-consumption.

1. Introduction

Although one can start using substances called drugs at any age, we know that most first experiences take place during adolescence. It seems that adolescence has always been characterized by an increasing desire for innovation, a search for new sensations, and the lure for transgression [By the way, all this is untrue….The very notion of the "adolescent" is very recent in Western history, and the concept of the teenager appeared only after World War 2] . Moreover, teenagers in our society are also relentlessly vigorously targeted as consumers of products. While the use of chemical substances, which are supposed to quickly enhance the sense of happiness and power, and which require little personal investment is encouraged [by whom?], the therapeutic discourse becomes increasingly more disqualified. Finally, adolescence is also a life-stage when concerns for health are few or even non-existent. Among the immense variety of substances circulating today, it seems that, over the past two decades, cannabis has become the drug of choice among teenager. They use it to identify with their peer group and as their distinctive symbol of generational membership. Although they also consume other substances such as ecstasy, LSD, cocaine, etc., we will mainly focus on their cannabis use, as it is not only the most representative of adolescents' drug habits, but also currently the most popular in the media.

2.Characteristics of Adolescence

2.1. Developmental Specificities of Adolescence

During adolescence, young people experience a peak in growth as well as important modifications of their identity and of the parameters that compose it --namely, emotions, challenges in familial and extra familial relations, in learning, etc. These changes often generate an intense questioning, and even a sense of chaos in all what they believed to know about themselves and their surrounding world.

In spite of these upheavals, teenagers remain disciplined by a system (school, in particular), which requires their concentration, curiosity, autonomy (for example in their homework) and a socially-induced growing preoccupation with performance at all costs. Learning is necessary to promote the development of their cognitive capacities, and the expansion of increasingly richer and complex neuronal connections. Those will enable them to acquire a whole array of aptitudes, which will also require them to use their cognitive endowment in the most possible efficient way.

Although present at any age, this neuronal plasticity is particularly important during childhood and adolescence, and any lack or reduction in stimulation can reduce the growth and the multiplication of these neuronal connections.

While growing up, teenagers not only acquire new capacities for self-reflection, but also learn how to use them, and to control their behaviors and emotions. During this period when their boiling neuronal system can trigger mood fluctuations and uncontrollable impulses, when spectacular synaptic reorganizations occur since the age of six and during the whole period of adolescence (accounting for the important increase of mood disorders, and for the exacerbation of the trouble that were present before this period of life) [1], adolescents must develop their aptitude to control these new sensations, and learn to integrate them into an acceptable social and relational functioning. This is very very unclear.

Often through trial and error, adolescents adapt their behaviors to that of their social environment, which allows them not only to extent their "nervous network", but also their social and relational ones, as these become progressively richer and extending beyond the family boundaries.

A new sense of belonging develops; peer groups become their source of identification and their major reference group, thus replacing the parents, who were their predominant model during infancy. Codes and rules change, and they affirm their membership in peer group by asserting their autonomy, sometimes through more or less serious transgressions of societal laws and cultural codes. Thus, their often-provoking dress codes, incorrect use of language, disrespect of parental instructions, discovering and experimenting with substances such as cannabis are actually included in the extension of adolescents' extra-familial social networks mentioned above.

2.2. Typology of Substance-Use During Adolescence

The last decade has witnessed a transformation in the ways young people use cannabis: first timers are progressively younger and quickly slip from recreational use to abuse, which often results in their dropping out.

Traditionally, young people and adults' substance use was classified as three types: substance use, substance abuse, addiction.

Substance use: "use is characterized by consumption of substances that does not involve complications or damages. This definition, which can lead to controversy, implies that there exists a consumption without risks --a socially regulated, accepted, and even valued substance that one uses for personal pleasure or convivial purposes." [2] The boundaries of the concept "use" are blurred because this definition does not distinguish between various categories of individuals who have similar patterns of use (car drivers, pregnant women, etc.)

Substance abuse: "abuse is characterized by the repetition of substance consumption, and the presence of observed social somatic, or legel damages (...) These damages can often be related to some of the abuser's psychological characteristics (i.e. impulsiveness, sensation seeking, transgression, etc.) that would explain both their increased consumption of toxic substances and their risk-seeking behaviors."

Dependence: "dependence on a substance is defined as psychopathological and behavioral tendencies that deviate from ?(Threaten? Endanger?) a person's usual functioning. In order to diagnose dependence, the usual signs of tolerance (the need to increases the doses of the substance in order to reach the same effects), and of weaning (physical syndrome occurring in case of deprivation of the substance), must be complemented by signs of compulsive craving for the substance, and the subject's inability to cease consumption in spite of its deleterious social and somatic consequence. (…) The label dependence rests thus less on the chemical properties of the substance than on the the experience it triggers in the person -- although this experience admittedly varies across substances. Each user finds in the substance of choice the specific effect s/he seeks (euphoria, stimulation, or sedation)."

Three other types of cannabis consumption can be identified, especially among young people: occasional, festive, self-therapeutic, and smash "anti thought" use (I count 4).

"First time" consumption generally occurs in peer groups where adolescents share a "joint." After the experimental phase, while many adolescents' use will remain festive or convivial, others, who are generally more vulnerable, will unfortunately use cannabis for its relaxing and hypnotic effects that soothe tension,,and help alleviate sleep disorder, or other problems. We call this type of use "self-therapeutic." (in the US, we say "self-medication") In this type of use, cannabis becomes indispensable for its benefits, even though there is no dependence to it, properly speaking. Still, signs of weaning can be present during periods of abstinence.

We can also distinguish between three types of daily consumption: moderated (3 to 5 joints, i.e. less than 1 gram), strong (5 to 6 joints, i.e. up to 1,2 gram) and intensive (more than 1,2 gram).

2.3. Risk Typologies

Numerous problems must be mentioned with regard to the typology of risks.

Risks Associated with School and Professional Learning

By reducing concentration and motivation, cannabis can threaten the capacity for learning that is crucial during adolescence. While we cannot be certain that these symptoms (in particular the "a-motivational" ones that we describe below) result from cannabis consumption, or pre-exist and partly explain it, an increasing number of researchers seem to support the second assumption. In other words, teenagers, who for genetic and environmental reasons, are more vulnerable than others, run a greater risk of over-consuming.

Age at First Consumption as a Worsening Factor

Some authors insist that the greatest vulnerability [to what?] is related to precocity of consumption. Indeed, Golub[3] and Perkonigg [4] suggest that the earlier an adolescent consumes cannabis, the greater the risks not only of abuse and/or dependence, but also of consumption of other illicit drugs. Early consumption also seems to increase the risk of the occurence of psychiatric pathologies, particularly when premorbid risk factors (schizoid personality...) are also present.

The Role of Biological Factors

As described above, while biological factors (i.e. synaptic reorganization) can interact with cannabis consumption and increase psychiatric risks (eating disorders, alcohol abuse, depressive symptoms, anxiety disorders, suicidal behavior, schizophrenia …) the role of cannabis consumption in the appearance of these disorders (which remain frequent during adolescence and early adulthood) remains uncertain.

The Emotional Impact of Cannabis Consumption

Physical and psychic changes affect the regulation of emotions.

During adolescence, and outside the (often protective) family environment, one is exposed to a wide array of new relationships whose intense emotional charges can be experienced as dangerous (break-up and relational disappointment, lack of acceptance, search for identity).

Intrafamilial relations also can be the source of conflicts and of disillusionment with the adult world, as adolescents might also have a difficult time integrating their new perceptions of the adult world, which they often see as meaningless and empty of ideals.

In such conditions, the consumption of cannabis can greatly enable the felt need to distance oneself from familiar objects of attachment and from the everyday world. Of course, adolescents first consume cannabis with friends, seeing this practice as a bonding ritual. However, when they start to consume it alone and on a daily basis, one also notes a reduction in, and even the disappearance of relational investments as well as divestment from those activities in which they once enthusiastically participated. Cannabis has thus the double effect of both gratifying teenagers' desires and urges for a relation of double dependence, and of providing a protective shell against external and internal stimulations [threats to the emerging self?]. In so doing, cannabis consumption provides the illusion of freedom while at the same time, masking one's increasing dependence on it.

3. Characteristics of the Substance

3.1. Cannabis, Origins and Pharmacology

The origins of the use of cannabis as a psychotropic substance go back to Antiquity. The plant itself, *"cannabis sativa"* Latin for hemp, was already cultivated more than 6,000 years ago in Asia.

In most societies, it was consumed for its psychoactive properties in therapeutic as well as in religious, political, or recreational contexts. Believed to faciliate the user's access to the divine realm, it was already used as a psychotropic substance in India more than 3,000 years ago.

Europe discovered cannabis following the return of the Crusaders and the Arab invasion. The widespread use of cannabis among Arab populations was supported by the religious Muslim prohibition against alcohol consumption. In 1800, Bonaparte was one of the first European to have prohibited his troops stationed in Egypt from consuming cannabis [for obvious reasons...ha ha...make love not war!!] . It was however used in France in recreational contexts. It was, for example, very popular in circles of artists such as the Hachichins' club in Paris, attended by Flaubert, Dumas, Baudelaire, and especially Theophile Gauthier.

In 1893, the Commission of Hemp in the United Kingdom, noted that "the abuse {this} drug can induce or maintain serious psychic disorders".

Influenced by "a prohibitionnist wave coming from the United States" [5], France prohibited the possession and and consumption of cannabis in 1953. In 1970, the public and private use of cannabis became punishable by law." [fascist pigs!]

From a pharmacological point of view, cannabis is composed of several substances of vegetable origin, most notably, cannabinoïds. Most important among them is delta-9-tétrahydrocannabinol (Δ^9THC), isolated in 1964 in Jerusalem. Delta-9-tétrahydrocannabinol is the principal psychoactive agent of cannabis. The distinctions among various seedlings hinges on their respective concentration of Δ^9THC. In France, below a concentration of 0,3 % of Δ^9THC, cannabis is considered as a plant of the "fiber" type. Beyond this level, it is considered a drug, whose cultivation is prohibited. Δ^9THC binds to CB1 (mainly central) and CB2 (primarily peripheral) receptors, which were respectively discovered in 1990 and 1993. In 1992, researchers discovered the anandamide --an endogenous compound, which can also bind to the two types of receptors. This discovery therefore also pointed at the existence of an endogenous cannaninoid system in the human organism.

These receptors are mainly located at the level of the cerebral anatomical structures that are implicated in memory and learning (cortex and hippocampus), psychomotor performances and driving coordination (basal ganglia and cerebellum), and in data processing systems associated with the perception of pain (peri-acqueducale gray surface, and dorsal horn of the spinal cord). To a lesser extent, they are also present at the level of the amygdala (control of emotions, anxiety, fear), and of the hypothalamus (endocrine system) as well as at the level of the nucleus accumbens (the reward system). On the other hand, the quasi absence of receptors at the level of the cerebral trunk could explain the absence of vital risks in the event of cannabis abuse. The highlighting of receptors CB2 at the level of the immune system as a whole would account for the immunomodulating effects of cannabinoïds.[6]

3.2. Different Uses

Cannabis can be consumed as "grass" or marijuana (containing the lowest level of Δ^9THC, approximately 5,5 %), as resin (7% average content), and as oil (up to a very high 60 %).

These last years, the content of 9THC continuously increased, reaching sometimes 22 % for grass, or 31 % for resin. These THC-enhanced substances are however still rare in Europe.

In the U.S., grass is typically smoked pure, while it is often mixed with tobacco in Western Europe (joints) In the US, a joint is pure grass, but never mixed with tobacco. Note also the increasing popularity of bongs. Note also that in the US, marijuana is also used in culinary preparations.

Resin or hashish takes the form of "barrettes" [bricks?]. It is smoked with tobacco (joints) or sometimes used in culinary preparations ("space cake," drinks). But it also smoked pure.

Oil is also smoked with tobacco, or mixed with food.

Inhalation produces a fast effect within a maximum of half an hour following the beginning of consumption, and with an average duration of 2 to 4 hours (if it's really good stuff). Ingestion has a slower, more progressive, and longer action, but less euphoric effects. (then why bother??)

3.3. Physiological and Toxic Effects

Cardiovascular Effects

Acceleration of the heartbeat and sometimes palpitations, lasting approximately 3 hours, and vasodilatation of the blood vessels with possibly orthostatic hypotension and headaches in the upright station.

Bronchopulmonary Effects

Bronchodilatation with facilitation of breathing in the hour which follows; inflammation of the bronchi.

Ocular Effects

Conjunctival Hyperhemy (redness of the eyes)
Mydriasis, more rarely
Sometimes visual disorders

Digestive Effects

Xerostomiasis
Increase in appetite
Sometimes vomiting and diarrhea

Pregnancy

When crossing the placental barrier, cannabis harms the development of the foetus (reduction in the growth, behavior anomalies).

Effects of Regular Cannabis Consumption on Health

At the Neuro-Cognitive Level

Deterioration of short-term memory.

Possibility of cerebral anomalies in cases of early consumption (before 16 years)

To date, neuro-imagery.techniques have revealed no neurotoxicity.

Nevertheless, it seems difficult to deny that THC could modify behavior by causing fine biological disordered states, which then deteriorate those cerebral systems responsible for the transmission of information. Fortunately, these effects are reversible.

At the Respiratory Level

Chronic consumption of cannabis causes disorders very similar to those induced by tobacco: cough and chronic bronchitis. The concentration of carcinogenic substances present in the smoke of cannabis is twice as high as in tobacco, with all the attendant risks of cancers of the respiratory and digestive tracks that it entails. A Tunisian study showed that the risk of lung cancer is eight times higher among cannabis users than among tobacco users [7].

At the Immunological Level

In vitro studies showed evidences of disturbances in the immune system. Accordingly, great care must be exercised when recommending cannabis as an analgesic to patients (cancer, AIDS) who already suffer from a weakened immune system.

At the Endocrine Level

Lastly, in vitro studies with rats also highlighted a reduction in testosterone secretion, testicle atrophies, disturbances in the production of sperm, and modification of sexual behavior in males (ouy youy, dis!), as well as disturbances in the ovulation cycle in females.

3.4. Effects and Psychic Risks

Acute Effects or Cannabic Intoxication

In the 19th century, the French mental specialist doctor Jacques-Joseph Moreau from Tours described in a poetic way the immediate psychic effects of cannabis. One could summarize them as follows: euphoria and wellbeing, excitation and thought dissociation, increased sensory perceptions, and errors in time and space perception.

However, individuals vary widely in terms of the level and sequence of these manifestations.

In general, the consumption of cannabis transforms the perception of the world, and includes distortion of self-image, and of temporal perception (lengthening of time), and increased intensity of sensory perceptions. Easy laughter, talkativeness, and satisfaction are some of the effects associated with cannabis-induced euphoria and well-being. The consumer simultaneously feels intellectual excitation and a feeling of calm and relief.

The effectsof cannabis on memory are important. They include deterioration of short-term memory, and difficulties of concentration. Thus, subjects experience difficulties remembering images, names, or words they saw or heard when they were under the influence of cannabis. Although these memory disorders can persist for several weeks after consumption has ceased, they are fortunately reversible.

An important reduction in motor coordination, and an increase in reaction time are also common, making driving under the influene of cannabis as dangerous as under the influence of alcohol. Importantly, the effects of cannabis on motor coordination last longer than alcohol, even though the subject is not conscious of the decline in his/her performance.

In contrast to its desired effects, cannabis can also produce less pleasant effects, such as sickness (a bit vague), sometimes accompanied by depressive ideas, or episodes of panic attacks (nearly 20 % of cannabis users will experience states of acute anxiety or panic attacks) [8]. Cases of cannabis-induced psychoses have also been reported, those seem to occur mainly among individuals whose consumption is substantial or chronic (in India and the Maghreb). It also seems that these "negative" effects occur particularly among people already displaying a pre-existing psychological vulnerability. "Cannabic psychosis" takes the form of confused or delirious states of paranoia, hallucinations, suicidal ideas, aggressiveness, and a weakening of psychomotor inhibition. Its prevalence is assessed at 0.1% of all consumers. It is most likely to appear during the intoxication phase or in the month following it, and is of short duration (less than 4 months). A neuroleptic treatment decreases its symptoms.

The Effects of Regular Cannabis Consumption on Mental Health and Social Development

The a-Motivational Syndrome

Derealization, a-pragmatism {what do you mean?}, apathy, difficulties to project oneself in the future, loss of energy, lack of interest, emotional numbing, reduction in intellectual communication skills, and lowered threshold of tolerance to frustration are the main parameters of this syndrome. Subjects are however typically aware of their passivity and withdrawal, and this syndrome is reversible with the discontinuation of consumption. [9]

However, since these symptoms are also observed in teenagers who suffer from depression and who do not consume cannabis, the causality between cannabis consumption and this a-motivational syndrome has been challenged. INSERM and other authors (the Scientific International Conference on Canabis, Brussels, 2002; Canadian Senate Special Comity on Illicit substances, 2002) have concluded that other emotional or psychosocial factors are not only as significant as cannabis consumption for the occurence of these symptoms, but that they could even trigger cannabis consumption.

One can easily understand that, together, these symptoms can have quite deleterious consequences with regard to school attendance, motivation and young consumers' learning capacities.

Consequence of Cannabis Consumption on Adolescents' Interpersonal Relationships

The consequences of cannabis consumption are important, especially in terms of parents-child relationships, and make family therapeutic work rather difficult. Members of the adolecent's milieu react differently to the problematic consumption, and these reactions partly influence the possibility of overtly talking about these problems and their possible aggravation. Thus, continuous denial or suspiciousness with ceaseless control, "enabling" behaviors (consisting of providing cannabis, excuses for absenteeism...), threats of total severing of the relations, or kicking the adolescent user out of the home are frequent and potentially harmful responses to his/her cannabis consumption. The parents' inconsistency that sometimes softens and sometimes exacerbates societal attitudes (ambiguous legality toward consumption or detention) contributes to the young consumers' experiencing the absence of clear boundaries. This experience in turn results in a sense of anguish or of distress, which will further increase their likelihood of consuming this substance.

The Aggravation of Psychiatric Symptoms

The aggravation of pre-existing or potential psychiatric symptoms in vulnerable patients also constitutes a growing concern for mental health professionals.

Relationship between Cannabis and Schizophrenia

Approximately 15 to 40 % of schizophrenic patients have experienced problems of abuse or dependence on cannabis during their life, versus 5,6 to 7,7 % in the general population. The reasons for their consumption are the same as those found in the general population: the search for euphoria, sociability, and sometimes for sedative or anti-depressant effects. It is also interesting to note that membership in a "community" of drug addicts may seem preferable to the label of mental patient. It seems that the worsening of schizophrenic symptoms caused by cannabis consumption is recognized today by a majority of clinicians.

Indeed, increases in hallucinations, delusions, frequencies and timing of relapses, admissions to emergency services, suicidal risks, and a reduction in compliance and social integration have all been noted. Nowadays, an increasing number of researchers hypothesize that cannabis may induce schizophrenia., and several recent studies [10] have confirmed that of cannabis consumption increases the risk of schizophrenia in predisposed individuals. This risk is positively correlated with the amount of intake and is expected to increase with precocity of consumption among predisposed individuals. Other studies suggest a certain level of similarity between genetic factors of schizophrenia and cannabis abuse, and observe more cannabis consumption among individuals who are, genetically, high-risk subjects for schizophrenia. Thus, in order to mitigate certain anomalies, current research efforts stress the close links existing between canabinoïds and dopaminergic systems with cannabis abuse and vulnerability to schizophrenia, since both lead to an increase of dopamine secretion.

Links between Depression and Cannabis

While many studies investigating these links are available, their interpretations are generally ambiguous and complex. Indeed, biases are numerous (difficulty in isolating depression as a criterion, retrospective character problems of memorization, insufficiently representative samples, short duration of studies...). We will distinguish here between two important issues, namely cannabis as causing depression and depression as causing cannabis dependency With regard to the former, most studies indicate only a modest contribution of cannabis to depression, and emphasize that the severity and precocity of cannabis intake increase the risks of cannabis-induced depression. On the other hand, the role of depression as a motivating factor for cannabis consumption is much more controversial. Whereas clinical observations indicate frequent mood aggravations caused by cannabis intake, longitudinal studies disconfirm this hypothesis.

Links with other Psychic Pathologies

Anxiety disorders are frequently associated with cannabis consumption, as its sedative property might hyopothetically be used for self medication. Thus, close to 1 out of five regular cannabis users presents an anxiety disorder[5].

If these two last associations (anxiety and depression disorder) have modest implications at the individual level, the widespread consumption of cannabis observed today is likely to inflate these consequences to society at large and to teenagers in particular, and will require clear information and preventive efforts.

Bulimia, a mainly feminine pathology, is also quite frequently associated with the consumption of cannabis in 15 to 45% of the cases. This comorbidity has important social and professional implications, and increases the importance of this disorder in comparison to the "pure" compulsive eaters. However, given the extreme variability of the results, they should be interpreted cautiously.

The association between the use of cannabis and suicidal risks also seems important, as the suicial risk is twice higer among cannabis users (abusive or not) than in the general population. When we consider that in France, approximately 40 000 young people attempted suicide (Inserm 2001) --and 800 of them succeeded--even a tiny increase in suicidal risk due to cannabis can have important implications for public health, and must therefore also be taken into account in prevention campaigns.

4. Epidemiology and at Risk Populations

4.1. Epidemiology

Over the last decade, we have witnessed a significant increase in cannabis consumption in the population at large, and especially among young adults.

The percentage of consumers varies across countries. In France, one out of three teenagers aged 15 to 19, and more than half of the the 18 year old have already consumed cannabis at least once. In Belgium also, one out of two young persons have tried cannabis before the age of 18. The United Kingdom and Ireland have a prevalence of consumption around 35 % among young people. These trends have been quite stable over the last few years, when compared to all other European countries where they continuously increase. Indeed, according to the European survey Espad [11] conducted among high school students, more than 36 % of 18 year old male teenagers admit having consumed cannabis at least ten times in 1999 versus 14 % in 1993.

According to certain studies (CFES)[12], it seems that experimenting with cannabis is most frequent between the ages of 15 and 34, with a peak around 20 (almost 60% of the subjects), with a prevalence among males (the male/female ratio is 1,3).[13].

More recent studies show that initiation to cannabis currently occurs between the ages 15 and 19, and adolescents younger than 15 account for only approximately 5% of new users. This age of first experimentation is rather similar to that of initiation to tobacco (14 years), and alcohol (13 years). Since we already know about the increased risk of consuming a variety of substances following experimentation with one, prevention efforts centered on these three problems appear more than justified.

Studies exclusively devoted to the issue of regular chronic consumption are much more scarce. An investigation within the framework of "Barometer Health" in 2000 (France), reveals that 20% of the 12-75 population have experimented with cannabis at least once (first consumption), 6 % are occasional users (from 1 to 9 times per annum), 4 % are repeated users (more than 10 times during the year but less than 10 times per month) and 3% are regular users (at least 10 times the last month). Focused research on the 18-25 age-group reveals that 14,6 % are regular consumers. The "Escapad" study [14] of 2000 reveals that, on average, 6,6% adolescent males aged 17 to 19, and 2,6 % female adolescents aged 17 are regular cannabis consumers. Female adolescents thus still remain a minority among consumers.

4.2. At Risk Population

Listening to young overconsummers' accounts [15] suggests that no factor can predict this behavior. The users originate from very diverse social backgrounds, live in quite different situations; their "first time" are different from each other, and do not seem to guide them toward either occasional or regular use of cannabis.

However, sociological studies reveal certain risk factors associated with regular consumption: father's high socio-professional level, parents living in different locations, and especially, early exposure to psychoactive substances such as tobacco and alcohol that adolescents later associate with polysubstance use. A sociological analysis of cannabis consumption shows that the age of experimentation --which peaks at around 20-- is mainly explained by the absence of age-specific social status markers. [16]

Genetic studies show that a genetic vulnerability predisposing to abuse or dependence on cannabis and other psychoactive substances does indeed exist, but manifests itself only in the presence of environmental and familial factors, which interact with individual ones. Those pertain especially to the the quality of the child's interaction with his or her environment and the quality of the development of his psychic structure.

If a parent is dependent on a particular substance, the risk of the child developing a problematic use of cannabis is approximately 5,8 times higher than in the normal population (in comparison, it is 4,2 higher for alcohol and 10 times higher for opiates). However, this risk is not solely explained by genetic factors but also by the simple fact of living and observing the practices of the addicted parent. In addition, the more a parent uses painkillers, anti-depressants, anti-anxiety or other substances that increase his or her sense of happiness or performance, the more the teenage child will turn to these substances when confronting stress or difficulties.

Discussing personality risks, Bergeret concluded that "there is not any psychic major and stable structure that is specific to addiction. Any mental structure can lead to addictive behaviors under certain emotional and relational conditions [...] addiction is an attempt to protect and regulate onseself against the deficiencies or the occasional flaws of the underlying structure in question"[17] One cannot thus predict the risk of consumption of or dependence on substances on the basis of personality traits.

5. Sociocultural Factors and the Evolution of Consumption

As we have just shown, cannabis is the substance of choice among teenagers, a finding that confers a diabolic aura to this substance, and adds to the typical lack of understanding that characterizes the relations between young and the adults. This distorted perception partly explains the much noisier ruckus around this substance than around alcohol, a quite harder but legal psychotropic substance, which has already been consumed at least once by approximately 90 % of the French population (versus 20 % for cannabis!), and which 25% men and 10% women aged 12 to 75 consume daily.

Nevertheless, one cannot help but wonder about the increased consumption of cannabis on a worldwide scale, and about the links between this increase and our current social system. First of all, in contrast to what most mass media assert, this increase did not really begin decades ago, but more precisely in the last 10 years --a period that witnessed an explosion in the supply of cannabis. This enormous increase in supply is partly explained by the increase of particularly prosperous cannabis cultures in Third World areas, where cannabis has a long tradition and strong economic motivations (for example in the Morocan Rif where the culture of cannabis constitutes the peasants' major source of income).

Considering the demand in Europe, this source of cannabis production will not easily dry up. One must also note the appearance in Europe and in the United States of a new genus of hydroponic and indoors cannabinoid plants (Skunk) that contain higher concentration of THC. ["Skunk" is something else…it's typically poor quality]. It thus seems obvious that the increase in demand created a more important, more accessible, more diversified, less expensive AND MORE POTENT supply.

Depending on one's model of society, one can also point at other reasons that explain this increase in consumption. In simple terms, the guiding principle, which organizes our society is the consumption imperative. When assessing individual and societal economic health, criterion of "productive capacities" has long been displaced by the "purchasing power" one. The media–orchestrated bombardment of messages that promote comfort as a must, and that promise miraculous solutions for every imaginable problem induce real "impulses to consume" products, which, we are told, will make us happy. Among young people, cannabis unsurprisingly also fulfills this function of immediate gratification. More alarmingly, our society does not only peddle products that are supposed to make us happy, but also painkillers in the broad sense of the term. As suffering and distress have become increasingly intolerable and unacceptable, we are ncreasingly encouraged to eliminate those inconvenient experiences as fast as possible, and effortlessly. The spectacular increase in the prescriptions of antidepressants these last years attests to this new psychocultural trend [see Gottschalk 2006, for an especially brilliant treatment of these trends] Cannabis fulfills these same needs. It also provides a temporary relief from suffering, at the cost of risking overconsumption and dependence.

Moreover, the increased frequency of addictive behavior among teenagers co-occur with an increase in other behavioral problems as well: impulsiveness, running away, violence, delinquence, suicide attempts, etc. According to Bergeret et al., this increase expresses an important distress in the population that revolves around dissatisfaction in terms of imagined ideals, dreams, and nonmaterial (only?) desires. As the ideals our society's media ceaselessly parade (money, success, beauty) seem empty and, in any case, inaccessible to most, teenagers react through these types of behavioral disorders (see also Merton's work on deviance and anomie).

While attempts to explain adults' lack of understanding with regard to cannabis consumption often mention the concept of generation gap, in contemporary society, confusion between generations seems to be the rule rather than the exception. The "open" dialogue between parents and children, the progressive weakening of the father's role and authority, and the fashionable trend of being "friends" with one's children, lead to a certain disappearance of conflicts, and induce young people to assert their sense of self by engaging in inadequate behaviors, such as consuming toxic substances (cannabis in particular), which, in turn, leads to many tensions and concerns.

Among their many concerns, adults tend to believe that their child's regular consumption of cannabis often masks the existence of deeper problems, and that early cannabis consumption can have considerable negative consequence for his her future.

Adults often seek to understand the core reason explaining why young people smoke, and are regularly frustrated in this endeavor because, to be strictly accurate, most of the time, there is none. Teenagers spend a lot of time outside the home, strike new friendships. On any particular day, a friend will offer the adolescent a joint, and the adolescent will see little reason to reject this offer. Thus, some are initiated by their peers, and others decide to experiment with it on their own. Some will not repeat this experience, and others will. Whatever the circumstances of the "first time", it is, before anything else, a symbolic act of transition from childhood to adolescence, of questioning parental authority, and of one's search for one's place in society. The joint is not a problem or a solution to a difficulty, and in any case, teenagers do not see it as a problem. This is why parents' framing of cannabis use as a form of self-therapy will only result in their children's refusal to talk. Encouraging young cannabis consumers to speak about their problems, without condemning them or pointing at cannabis' therapeutic effects will be a much more fruitful approach to help them assess the influence of cannabis on these problems.

Lastly, one of the most frequently heard concerns voiced by adult society pertains to the "slippery slope" theory –or the belief that the consumption of cannabis is the first step in a downward spiral leading towards the use of harder drugs. According to research, there is indeed a risk of polyuse among young consumers, who developped very precociously addictive potentials. Living in an environment where the use of drugs is normal also constitutes a main entrance to poly-substance addiction. Because these young people often endure a harsh environment, where suffering is often present, it is these conditions, not cannabis per se, that can lead them to consume increasingly powerful and destructive substances.

It is also true that dealers who sell cannabis often also sell other substances. While the availability of these more dangerous substances can facilitate their experimentation, we cannot offer any firm conclusion about the direct links between cannabis and other substances (the "slippery slope"). Besides, the existence of "coffee-shops" in the Netherlands, which can legally deliver small amounts of cannabis (5 grammes/day), constitutes a response to this theory and is a pragmatic attempt to prevent young users from participating in the cannabis underground networks as well as limit their exposure to other and more toxic drugs .

6. Conclusion : Assessing the Risk Associated with Consumption

6.1. When Should We Start Worrying? What Should We Do in the Face of Consumption?

Today, parents' concerns are no longer related to the real existence of consumption but to the anticipatory fear that their child might be exposed to cannabis, might try it out, and become a "first timer." However, we saw that currently, the majority of young people will have experimented with cannabis at least once in their life, and most of those, before the age of 18. 18. While parental anticipatory anxiety is certainly justified by the extent of the phenomenon, it risks to create additional tensions and a larger gap between the generations, i.e. between young people who do not see any evil in smoking a joint from time to time, since all their friends do, and parents who sometimes display disproportionate stress.

Let us keep in mind that if overconsumers indeed exist, they still represent only a tiny minority of consumers. They often suffer greatly, but do not represent all users.

Consumption becomes worrisome when it is no longer occasional or festive, when young consumers devote more time and money to it, when they stop socializing, and experience falling grades at school as result of increased consumption. While these changes can be indicators of the gravity of the phenomenon, they can also result from a psychiatric disorder or an important psychological distress. To blame all emerging problems and behavioral changes to cannabis would run the risk of overlooking the reality of suffering a young person might be experiencing.

We should also be cautious not to assume "experimentation" when the behavior under consideration might be more serious. Being attentive without becoming intrusive remains an important means of detecting a skid towards regular consumption. Nurturing a climate of trust should also encouage young people to discuss their concerns with a problematic consumption, and thus start confronting the problem at an earlier stage. Rather than imposing our own interpretation of the problem on them, we should remember that reassuring them of our availability and concern is sometimes the only message they hope for before they can formulate a real desire of help.

While social workers can develop this attitude, it is the parents who are especially the first line of defense. Although children might often reject their help, they almost always recognize their essential importance once the crisis has been resolved.

Until they become self-aware of the imbalance cannabis causes in their lives, young people will, for a long time, often deny any link between the difficulties they encounter and their consumption. Often, they also come to realize that the cost/benefit, pleasure/displeasure balance is no longer advantageous, that their consumption harmed relations with family and friends, or that they have too frequent problems with the police. Confronting these negative outcomes, they may then decide to change their behavior –sometimes successfully, and often with difficulties. They often associate ceassation of cannabis use with leaving a certain social environment that is often tied with delinquency or marginality. When consumption took them this far afield, they are likely to experience difficulties with the project of rebuilding a new sense of self, of leaving the social network that led to delinquency or marginality, and of coming to terms with the years they lost to cannabis, especially the school years.

It is in this period of awakening that young people will especially need support.

From a psychological point of view, one can offer teenagers one-on-one conversations in order to assess the difficulties they are encountering and also to help them develop strategies that will prevent a relapse.

Helping the consumer's family is also essential, as it will enable to identify the dysfunctions that might have prompted the teenager's consumption, and those that resulted from it.

Finally, various forms of social intervention might also be important, particularly in those cases where consumption resulted in school dropout, delinquency, and marginalization.

6.2. Strategies of Information, Prevention, Reduction of Risk and Health Care

Considering the complex phenomenon of youth's addiction to cannabis, any simple solution runs the risk of quickly becoming simplistic, reductionist, moralistic, ideological, and even hypocritical. It is also fairly obvious that the Law alone will not solve this problem. Regardless of the different legal provisions regulating cannabis use in different Western countries, the mere fact that the number of cannabis consumers is constantly increasing attests to their shortcomings and impotence. While the existence of a legal framework is clearly useful, one should not try to solve this problem by invoking a kneejerk call for law and order.

As we have argued, the complexity of dependence problems cannot be reduced to particular characteristics of the concerned population, but must also include the illicit and illegal nature of most drugs.

To complicate matters further, the problems of addiction are only in rare cases limited to the use of one single substance, and very frequently co-occur with other nonpharmacological addictions, such as pathological gambling and, in particular, addiction to the Internet. In light of these patterns, we have no choice but emphasize that this problem is not limited to cannabis, ecstasy, cocaine, LSD or heroin, but that it also --and chiefly--includes tobacco and alcohol, which, lest we forgot, are legal substances. Returning to teenagers' addictions, the menu they can choose from thus includes cannabis, which is prohibited but widespread; alcohol, which is authorized and often glamorized; and tobacco, which is legal but demonized. *This triad being hot on the heels of abuse of primarily psychotropic and antalgic medical legal drugs*. [unclear] Fortunately, therefore, cannabis presently lags behind synthetic drugs such as cocaine, whose use is however rapidly growing, LSD and other hallucinogens, as well as heroin, which has expreienced a loss of popularity, at least in its "junkie" version.

Each era and society defines its "taboos" according to moral (personal freedom, dignity etc...), medical (physical and psychic damages) and legal (delinquency...) criteria. The political framing of dependence falls under this ethical tension between moral, medical, and legal considerations. A coherent policy with regard to health and dependence on substances, must imperatively seek a balance between these three fundamental criteria. This balance is however difficult to reach, particularly because of the contradictory nature of the unstable foundations of the taboos pertaining to drugs. In contrast to alcohol, the efforts invested in distinguishing between different types of uses are relatively fruitless with regard to recreational drugs *which social representations forecast the worst, even exclusively, the worst. [*unclear]

Indeed, it is in the name of this "worst medical forecast" and of concerns for public health that these substances are prohibited, whereas other poisons "of a better company" [?] like alcohol and tobacco are (still!) authorized. Overall, as you must have understood by now, there is a gap between the social representations of the "junkies" and the daily reality of users, particularly adolescents. Lastly, branding all illegal drugs with the same "illicit" label is likely to lump together cannabis --an altogether relatively not very toxic substance– with stimulant "speeders" such as cocaine, hallucinogenic "smashers" such as LSD, or "cooling" opiates such as heroin. This careless grouping cannot help but reinforce the lay person's confusion and upset with regard to drugs. Regardless of the real dangers these substances pose, the "drug problem" has been gradually constructed in a way that is guaranteed to fan the flames of fear and insecurity. As sociologist François Alain d' Ehrenberg suggests [18] people's attitude towars drugs in our society is 'radicalizing' in terms of the traditional dilemma of modern freedom between the right to treat one's body as one wishes [?], and the duty to belong to society, quartering users between disease and delinquency [?]. Currently, no thanks to fear and confusion, it is still the image of the cannabis user as a delinquent that predominates. Examining the budgets of the majority of Western countries, one will notice that approximately 55 % of the resources are allotted to repression, 40 % to health policies, 4 % to prevention, and a very small percentage to research. Thus, much remains to be accomplished. While we do not promote decreasing the repression of what should be be repressed, we do advocate increasing the resources invested in research (in the end, one can only act on the basis of full knowledge of the facts), information gathering (as neutrally and objectively as possible) on potential users, parents, teachers, migrants and policies, on reduction of risks, and care in the physical, psychic, and systemic fields. In order to be an effective tool stimulating the subject's autonomy, the legal framework must be clear. As one us (Prof. N. Zdanowicz [19]) wrote on several occasion with regard to dependence and other health disorders, it is important that teenagers realize that their health is too important to entrust to others.

7. REFERENCES

[1] Stahl SM. Psychopharmacologie essentielle. In *Médecine Sciences*. Flammarion, Paris, 2002.

[2] Phan O., Cornos M., Girardon N., Nezelof S., Jeammet P. Abus et dépendance au cannabis à l'adolescence. EMC (Elsevier SAS, Paris), *Psychiatrie/Pédopsychiatrie* 2005. 37-216-G-40.

[3] Golub A, Bruce DJ. The shifting importance of alcohol and marijuana as gateway substances among serious drug abusers. *J. Stud. Alcohol.* 1994 ; 55 : 607-14

[4] Perkonigg A, Lieb R, Höfler M, Schuster P, Sonntag H, Wittchen HU. Patterns of cannabis use, abuse and dependence over time ; incidence, progression and stability in a sample of 1228 adolescents. *Addiction.* 1999 ; 94 : 1663-78

[5] Chollet-Przednowed E., Cannabis : *le dossier,* Gallimard, Paris, 2003

[6] Reynaud Michel (sous la direction de) ; *Addictions et psychiatrie ;* Masson, Paris, 2005

[7] Hsairi M., Anchour N., Zouari B., Facteurs étiologiques du cancer bronchique primitif en Tunisie. *La Tunisie médicale.* 1997, 71 : p. 265-268

[8] Dervaux A., Kanit M., Laqueille X., Cannabis : attention aux comorbidités. *Rev. Prat.,* 2001, 540 : p.1163-1166.

[9] Palazzolo Jérôme, Fumer du cannabis : quels risques ? *Cerveaux and Psycho*, 2006, 15 : p74-79.

[10] Warner LA, Kessler RC, Hugues M et coll. Prévalence and correlates of drug use and dependance in the United States. *Arch. Gen. Psychiatry.* 1995, 52 : 219-29

[11] Arsenault L., Cannon M., Poulton R., Murray R., Caspi A., Moffitt T.E., Cannabis use in adolescence and risk for adult psychosis : longitudinal prospective stud. *Br. Med. J.,* 2002, 325: p.1212-1213.

[12] Van Os J., Bak M., Hanssen M., Bijl R.V., De Graaf R., Verdoux H., Cannabis use and psychosis: a longitudinal population-based study, *Psychol. Med.,* 2003, 33: p. 23-32

[13] Zammit S., Allebeck P., Andreasson S., Lundberg I., Lewis G., Self reported cannabis use as a risk factor for schizophrenia in Swedish conscripts of 1969: historical cohort stuffy. *Br. Med. J.,* 2002, 325: p. 1199-1201.

[14] ESPAD (European School Survey Project on Alcohol and Other Drugs) Choquet M., Ledoux S., Hassier C., Beck F., Peretti-Watel P., Consommations de substances psychoactives chez les 14-18 ans scolarisés (Inserm, OFDT, MENRT) : premiers résultats de l'enquête Espad 1999, évolution 1993-1999. *Tendances,* février 2000, n°6

[15] CFES (Comité français d'éducation pour la santé), aujourd'hui INPES (Institut national de prévention et d'éducation pour la santé), Baromètre santé 2000

[16] Beck F., Legleye S., Peretti-Watel P., *Baromètre santé.* 2000

[17] ESCAPAD (Enquête santé et consommation au cours de la journée de préparation à la Défense) Beck F., Legleye S., Peretti-Watel P., Regards sur la fin de l'adolescence. Consommation de produits psychoactifs dans l'enquête Escapad 2000, OFDT, décembre 2000

[18] Sous la direction de Descamps Luc et Hayez Cécile, Génération cannabis, paroles de jeunes, Paroles d'experts, L'Harmattan, Paris, 2005

[19] Aquatias S., Maillard I., Zoman M., Faut-il avoir peur du Haschisch ? *Syros,* 1999, p 224

[20] Bergeret J. Aspects économiques du comportement d'addiction. In Le psychanalyste à l'écoute du toxicomane. Dunod, Paris, 1981

[21] Zdanowicz N., Janne P., Reynaert Ch. Comparaison des attentes d'étudiants "sains" et "en souffrance" par rapport à leur famille. *Ann. Méd-psychol.* 2002 ; 160 : 130-137

[22] A. Ehrengerg. Drogues : éthique et politique des drogues. In Dictionnaire d'éthique et philosophie morale, tome 1, sous la direction de Monique Canto-Sperber. Puf, Quadrige, dico poche, Paris 2004

INDEX

A

D

E

F

G

H

I

N

O

P

T

U

V

W

X

Y